Radiology
Lecture Notes

Radiology
Lecture Notes

Pradip R. Patel

Consultant Radiologist
Kingston Hospital
London, UK

Fourth Edition

First edition awarded BMA Book Award

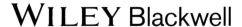

Registered Office(s)
John Wiley & Sons, Inc., 111 River Street, Hoboken, NJ 07030, USA
John Wiley & Sons Ltd, The Atrium, Southern Gate, Chichester, West Sussex, PO19 8SQ, UK

Editorial Office
9600 Garsington Road, Oxford, OX4 2DQ, UK

For details of our global editorial offices, customer services, and more information about Wiley products visit us at www.wiley.com.

Wiley also publishes its books in a variety of electronic formats and by print-on-demand. Some content that appears in standard print versions of this book may not be available in other formats.

Library of Congress Cataloging-in-Publication Data

Names: Patel, Pradip, author.
Title: Lecture notes. Radiology / Pradip Patel, Kingston Hospital,
    Woodlands, Kingston, UK.
Description: Fourth edition. | Hoboken : Wiley, 2020. | Series: Lecture
    notes | Includes bibliographical references and index.
Identifiers: LCCN 2020001869 (print) | LCCN 2020001870 (ebook) | ISBN
    9781119550341 (paperback) | ISBN 9781119550334 (adobe pdf) | ISBN
    9781119550372 (epub)
Subjects: LCSH: Radiography, Medical–Outlines, syllabi, etc.
Classification: LCC RC78.17 .P385 2010 (print) | LCC RC78.17 (ebook) |
    DDC 616.07/572–dc23
LC record available at https://lccn.loc.gov/2020001869
LC ebook record available at https://lccn.loc.gov/2020001870

Cover Design: Wiley
Cover Image: Courtesy of Pradip R. Patel; © piranka/Getty Images

Set in 8.5/11pt Utopia by SPi Global, Pondicherry, India
Printed and bound in Singapore by Markono Print Media Pte Ltd

10 9 8 7 6 5 4 3 2 1

Contents

List of contributors

Chapter 1
Dr Patricia Marin Crespo, Consultant Radiologist, Kingston Hospital, UK

Chapter 2
Dr Aghi Srikanthan, Consultant Radiologist, Kingston Hospital, UK

Chapter 3
Dr Vin Majuran, Consultant Radiologist, Kingston Hospital, UK

Chapter 4
Dr Sarah Evans, Consultant Radiologist, Kingston Hospital, UK

Chapter 5
Dr Ramesh Yella, Consultant Radiologist, Kingston Hospital, UK

Chapter 6
Dr Nevin Wijisekera, Consultant Radiologist, Kingston Hospital, UK

Chapter 7
Dr Nim Mangat, Consultant Radiologist, Kingston Hospital, UK

Chapter 8
Dr Pradip R. Patel, Consultant Radiologist, Kingston Hospital, UK

Chapter 9
Dr Bijan Heydati, Consultant Radiologist, Kingston Hospital, UK

Chapter 10
Dr Charlotte Whittaker, Consultant Radiologist, Kingston Hospital, UK

Chapter 11
Dr Derek Svasti-Salee, Consultant Radiologist, Kingston Hospital, UK

Chapter 12
Dr Pradip R. Patel, Consultant Radiologist, Kingston Hospital, UK

Chapter 13
Dr Pradip R. Patel, Consultant Radiologist, Kingston Hospital, UK

About the companion website

This book is accompanied by a companion website:

www.wiley.com/go/patel/radiology

The website includes:

- Self-assessment exercises to accompany each book chapter
- Chapter based exercises with further examples and images

Note: The website should be live by December 2020.

Introduction

Recent technological advances have produced a bewildering array of complex imaging techniques and procedures. The basic principle of imaging, however, remains the anatomical demonstration of a particular region and related abnormalities, the principal imaging modalities being:

- **plain X-rays**: utilizes a collimated X-ray beam to image the chest, abdomen, skeletal structures, etc.;
- **fluoroscopy**: a continuous X-ray beam produces a moving image to monitor examinations such as barium meals, barium enemas, etc.;
- **ultrasound (US)**: employs high-frequency sound waves to visualize structures in the abdomen, pelvis, neck and peripheral soft tissues;
- **computed tomography (CT)**: obtains cross-sectional computerized densities and images from an X-ray beam/detector system;
- **magnetic resonance imaging (MRI)**: exploits the magnetic properties of hydrogen atoms in the body to produce images;
- **nuclear medicine (NM)**: acquires functional as well as anatomical details by gamma radiation detection from injected radioisotopes.

Contrast media

Contrast agents are substances that assist visualization of some structures during the above techniques, working on the basic principle of X-ray absorption, thereby preventing their transmission through the patient. The most commonly used are barium sulphate to outline the gastrointestinal tract, and organic iodine preparations; the latter widely used intravenously in CT for vascular and organ enhancement. Contrast agents can also be introduced into specific sites, for example:

- *arteriography*: the arterial system;
- *venography*: the venous system;
- *myelography*: spinal theca;
- *cholangiography*: the biliary system;
- *hysterosalpingography*: uterus;
- *arthrography*: joints;
- *sialography*: salivary glands.

The possibility of an allergic reaction exists with iodinated contrast media, an increased risk noted in those with a history of allergy, bronchospasm and cardiac disease, as well as in the elderly, neonates, diabetics or patients with multiple myeloma.

- *Minor reactions*: nausea, vomiting, urticarial rash, headache.
- *Intermediate reactions*: hypotension, bronchospasm.
- *Major reactions*: convulsions, pulmonary oedema, cardiac arrhythmias, cardiac arrest.

Drug therapy should be readily available to treat reactions, for example:

- urticaria: chlorphenamine or other antihistamines;
- pulmonary oedema: furosemide i.v.;
- convulsions: diazepam i.v.;
- bronchospasm: hydrocortisone i.v. and bronchodilators such as salbutamol;
- anaphylactic reactions: adrenaline s.c. or i.v.

Radiation protection

All individuals receive natural background radiation but diagnostic tests now account for the largest source of exposure and every effort at reduction must be made. Although ionizing radiation is deemed to be potentially hazardous, the risks should be weighed in the context of benefits to the patient.

- Doses should be kept to a minimum and a radiological investigation performed only if management is going to be affected. Consideration should be given to the radiation dose to the patient for each specific investigation. CT, barium and radionuclide studies are high-dose examinations, whereas plain films of the extremities and chest X-rays are typically low dose.

Radiology: Lecture Notes, Fourth Edition. Pradip R. Patel.
© 2020 John Wiley & Sons Ltd. Published 2020 by John Wiley & Sons Ltd.
Companion website: www.wiley.com/go/patel/radiology

- The fetus is particularly sensitive, especially in the first trimester with possible induction of carcinogenesis or fetal malformation. A menstrual history obtained in a woman of reproductive age, and if necessary a pregnancy test, will prevent accidental fetal exposure to radiation.
- Clear requests to the radiology department, with relevant clinical details, aids in the selection of the most appropriate views or investigations.
- Discussion of complex cases with a radiologist may help in choosing the most relevant study or examination.
- Unnecessary examinations should be avoided, for example repeat chest X-rays for resolution of pneumonic consolidation at less than weekly intervals, or preoperative chest X-rays in young patients.
- Ultrasound and MRI, because of the lack of ionizing radiation, are the preferred imaging modalities where clinically indicated.

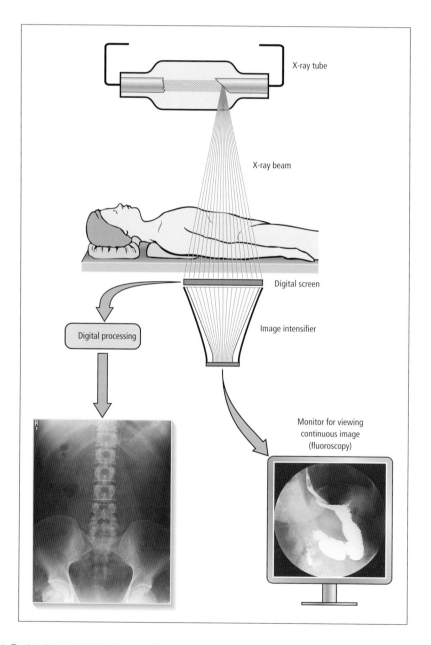

Figure 1.1 Basic principles of plain films and fluoroscopy.

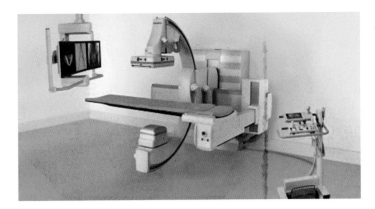

Figure 1.2 Digital plain film and fluoroscopy equipment.

Plain films and fluoroscopy

Conventional radiography

X-rays are part of the electromagnetic spectrum, emitted as a result of bombardment of a tungsten anode by free electrons from a cathode. Hard copy plain films are produced by their passage through the patient and exposing a radiographic film.

Bone absorbs most radiation, causing least film exposure, thus the developed film appears white. Air absorbs least radiation, causing maximum film exposure, so the film appears black. Between these two extremes a large differential tissue absorption results in a grey-scale image. The majority of plain films are now performed with digital radiography and conventional plain films are infrequently used.

Digital radiography

In digital radiography, the basic principles are the same but a digital screen replaces the X-ray film. The tissue absorption characteristics are computer analysed and the image is visualized on a monitor. CT, MRI and ultrasound are already available in digital format; with the rapid introduction of digital plain-film radiography, radiological departments are now filmless (picture archival and communication system, PACS). The principal advantages of digital radiography are:

- significant reduction in radiation exposure;
- digital enhancement ensures all images are of an adequate quality;
- transfer of images out of the radiology department to other sites;
- elimination of storage problems associated with conventional films;
- no hard copy films;
- rapid retrieval of previous images and reports for comparison;
- ease of availability of examinations to clinicians.

Plain film images are particularly useful for:

- chest;
- abdomen;
- skeletal system: trauma, spine, joints, degenerative, metabolic and metastatic disease.

Fluoroscopy/screening

Fluoroscopy is the term used when a continuous low-power X-ray beam is passed through the patient to produce a dynamic image that can be viewed on a monitor. Many different procedures, such as barium studies of the gastrointestinal tract, arteriography and interventional procedures, are monitored and carried out with the aid of fluoroscopy.

Ultrasound

Ultrasound employs high-frequency sound waves, produced by a piezo-electric crystal in a transducer. The waves travel through the body, and are reflected back variably, depending on the different types of tissue encountered. The same transducer, as well as transmitting ultrasound, receives the reflected sound and converts the signal into an electric current; this is subsequently processed into a grey-scale picture. A moving image is obtained as the transducer is advanced across the body (real-time ultrasound). Sections can be obtained in any plane and

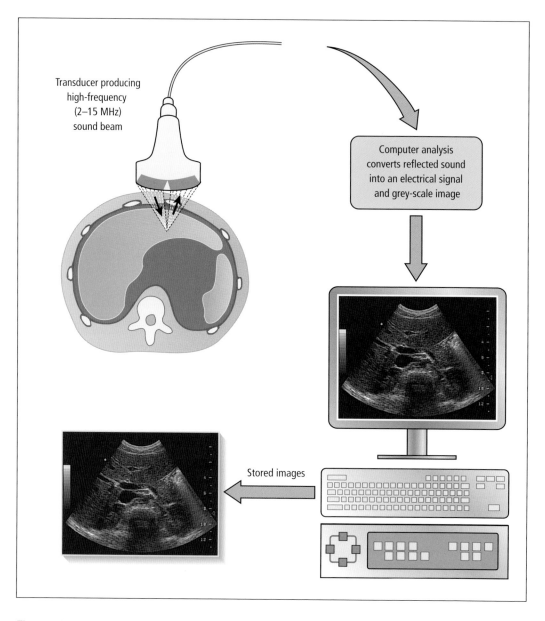

Figure 1.3 Basic principles of ultrasound.

viewed on a monitor. Bone and air are poor conductors of sound, thus there may be inadequate visualization, whereas fluid has excellent transmission properties.

Doppler ultrasound

Doppler ultrasound is a technique to examine moving structures in the body. Blood flow velocities are measured using the principle of a shift in reflected sound frequency produced from moving structures. It is utilized for:

- assessment of cardiac chambers and heart valves;
- arterial flow studies, especially carotids and peripheral vascular disease;
- venous flow studies for detection of deep vein thrombosis.

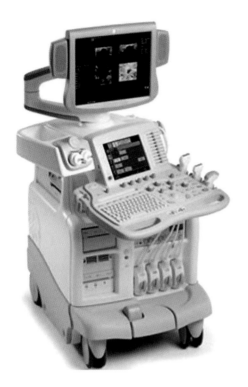

Figure 1.4 Ultrasound machine with differing frequency probes ranging from 5–20 MHz. Specialist ones include transvaginal, transrectal and musculoskeletal probes.

Uses
- Brain: Imaging the neonatal brain.
- Thorax: Confirms pleural effusions and pleural masses.
- Abdomen: Visualizes liver, gallbladder, pancreas, kidneys, etc.
- Pelvis: Useful for monitoring pregnancy, uterus and ovaries.
- Peripheral: Assesses thyroid, testes and soft-tissue lesions.

Advantages
- Relatively low cost of equipment.
- Non-ionizing and safe.
- Scanning can be performed in any plane.
- Can be repeated frequently, for example pregnancy follow-up.
- Detection of blood flow, cardiac and fetal movement.
- Portable equipment can be taken to the bedside for ill patients.
- Aids biopsy and drainage procedures.

Disadvantages
- Operator dependent.
- Inability of sound to cross an interface with either gas or bone causes unsatisfactory visualization of underlying structures.
- Scattering of sound through fat produces poor images in obesity.

Computed tomography

CT involves passage of a collimated X-ray beam through the patient to obtain images of thin transverse sections of the head and body. A sensitive detection system with photomultiplier tubes is employed, with the X-ray tube rotating around the patient during each cycle. An image is obtained by computer processing of the digital readings from the photomultiplier tubes and analysis of the absorption pattern of each tissue. Absorption values are expressed on a scale of +1,000 units for bone, the maximum absorption of the X-ray beam, to −1,000 units for air, the least absorbent.

Each image represents a section through the body, the thickness being varied from 1 to 10 mm. Tissues lying above or below this slice are not imaged and a series of slices is taken to cover a particular region. Rapid sequences can be obtained, with the thorax and abdomen imaged in a few seconds.

The CT image consists of a matrix of picture elements (pixels), the slice thickness giving the volume component (voxel). Each voxel represents the attenuation value of the X-ray beam at that particular point in the body.

Oral contrast is used to outline the gastrointestinal tract, and intravenous contrast to delineate the vascular system and to study organ enhancement in various pathological conditions.

Uses
- Any region of the body can be scanned: brain, neck, abdomen, pelvis and limbs.
- Staging primary tumours such as colon and lung for secondary spread, to determine operability or a baseline for chemotherapy.
- Radiotherapy planning.
- Exact anatomical detail when ultrasound is not successful.
- Vascular anatomy such as coronary arteries.

Advantages
- Good contrast resolution.
- Precise anatomical detail.

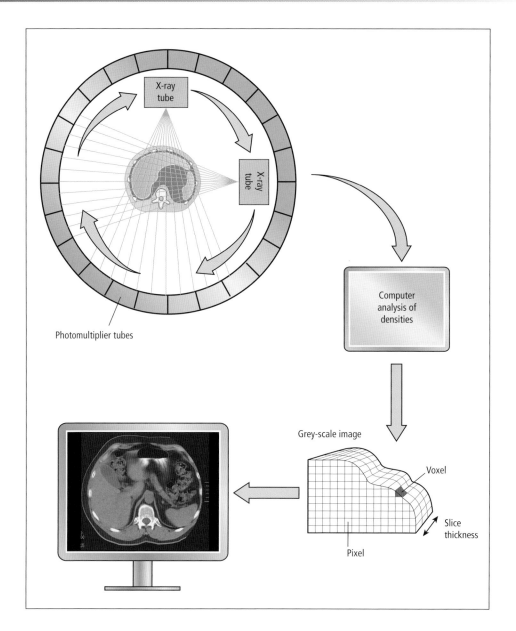

Figure 1.5 Basic principles of CT.

- Rapid examination technique, so valuable for ill patients.
- Good diagnostic images are obtained in obese patients as fat separates the abdominal organs, unlike ultrasound.

Disadvantages
- High dose of ionizing radiation for each examination.
- High cost of equipment and scan.
- Bone artefacts in brain scanning, especially the posterior fossa, degrade images.

- Scanning mostly restricted to the transverse plane, although reconstructed images can be obtained in other planes.

Magnetic resonance imaging

MRI produces images of the body by utilizing the magnetic properties of certain nuclei, principally those of

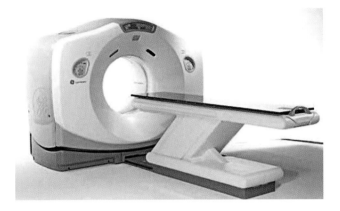

Figure 1.6 CT scanner.

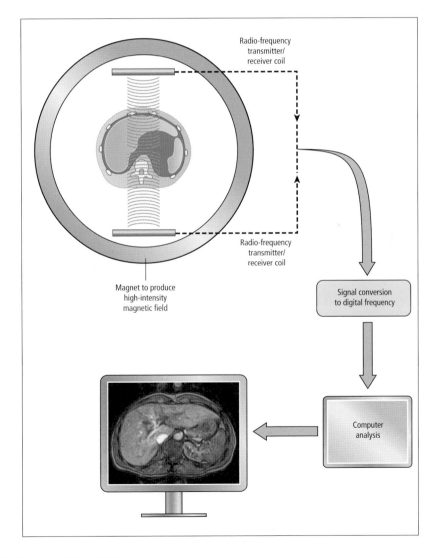

Radio-frequency
transmitter/
receiver coil

Radio-frequency
transmitter/
receiver coil

Magnet to produce
high-intensity
magnetic field

Signal conversion
to digital frequency

Computer
analysis

Figure 1.7 Basic principles of MRI.

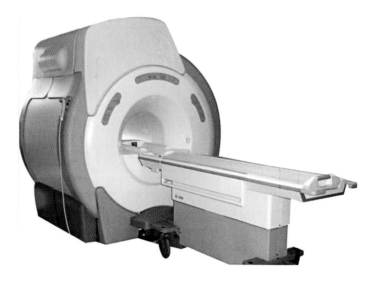

Figure 1.8 MRI scanner.

hydrogen in water molecules. The patient is placed in the scanner tunnel and subjected to a high-intensity magnetic field. This forces the hydrogen atom nuclei to align with the magnetic field. A pulse of radio-frequency applied to these nuclei then displaces them from their position; when the pulse ceases, they return to their original state, releasing energy (in the form of a radio-frequency signal). Computer analysis processes this energy into a digital signal, with conversion to a grey-scale image. Hence, the basic principle of MRI is a study of the response of magnetized tissue to a pulse of radio-frequency, whereby pathological tissue returns different signals compared to normal.

Uses
- Central nervous system (CNS): technique of choice for brain and spinal imaging.
- Musculoskeletal: accurate imaging of joints, tendons, ligaments and muscular abnormalities.
- Cardiac: imaging with gating techniques related to the cardiac cycle enables the diagnosis of many cardiac conditions.
- Thorax: assessment of vascular structures in the mediastinum.
- Abdomen: abdominal organs are well visualized, surrounded by high signal from surrounding fat.
- Pelvis: staging of prostate, bladder and pelvic neoplasms.

Advantages
- Can image in any plane – axial, sagittal or coronal.
- Non-ionizing and hence believed to be safe to use.
- No bony artefacts due to lack of signal from bone.
- Excellent anatomical detail, especially of soft tissues.
- Visualizes blood vessels without contrast: magnetic resonance angiography (MRA).
- Intravenous contrast utilized much less frequently than CT.

Disadvantages
- High operating costs.
- Poor images of lung fields.
- Inability to show calcification with accuracy.
- Fresh blood in recent haemorrhage not as well visualized as by CT.
- MRI more difficult to tolerate with examination times longer than CT.
- Contraindicated in patients with pacemakers, metallic foreign bodies in the eye and arterial aneurysmal clips (may be forced out of position by the strong magnetic field).

Nuclear medicine

Radionuclide imaging is a valuable diagnostic tool, the principal modality that examines abnormal physiology of the body in preference to anatomical detail. Technetium-99m is the commonest isotope used, and by tagging with certain substances, a particular region of interest can be targeted.

Positron emission tomography (PET)

PET uses positron-emitting isotopes, many short-lived and cyclotron produced. These agents include

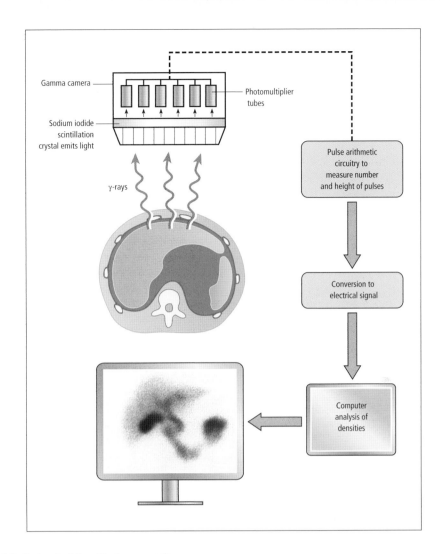

Figure 1.9 Basic principles of isotope scanning.

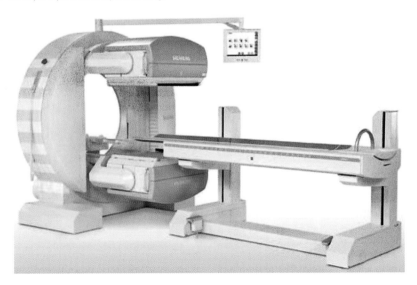

Figure 1.10 Nuclear medicine scanner.

Table 1.1 Typical applications of isotopes.

Anatomical area	Agent	Application
Respiratory tract	Tc99m microspheres Krypton, DTPA	Perfusion and ventilation scanning for diagnosis of pulmonary embolus
Cardiovascular	Thallium-201 Tc99m MIBI	For infarct imaging as it accumulates in normal myocardium showing a defect corresponding to infarcts
Gastrointestinal	Na pertechnetate and Tc99m-labelled WBCs	Studies to detect Meckel's diverticulum and inflammatory bowel conditions
Liver and spleen	Tc-labelled sulphur colloid	Reticuloendothelial uptake to image focal abnormalities
Biliary system	Tc99m HIDA	Useful in cholecystitis and obstruction, as isotope uptake in liver is excreted in bile
Urinary tract	DMSA MAG3	Studies of renal functional and anatomical abnormalities
Skeletal	Tc-labelled phosphonates	Uptake at sites of increased bone turnover, e.g. tumours and arthritis
Thyroid	Iodine-131 or Tc99m	Assessing focal nodules
Parathyroid	Sestamibi protein labelled with Technetium 99	May visualize adenomas

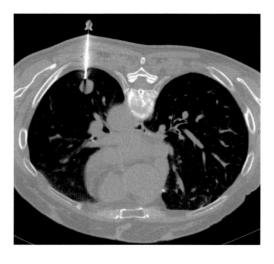

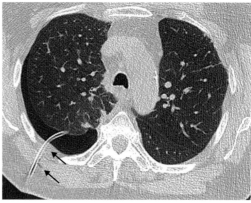

Figure 1.12 Insertion of a chest drain (arrows) under CT control for a pneumothorax.

Figure 1.11 A biopsy needle has been inserted under CT control into a lung nodule for histology samples.

radioactive oxygen, carbon and nitrogen but the commonest in use is fluorodeoxyglucose (FDG), a glucose analogue, indicating tissue metabolic activity in the detection of tumours or secondary deposits. It is often combined with a CT to give anatomical as well as functional information. Accurate studies of blood flow and metabolism are also possible using these tracers.

Interventional radiology

Respiratory tract

Lung biopsy

A needle is inserted directly into the lung or pleural mass and tissue taken for microbiological or histological analysis. The procedure may be performed under fluoroscopy or CT.

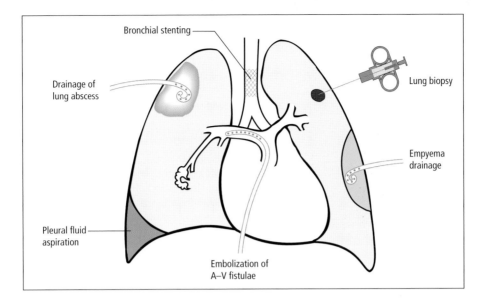

Figure 1.13 Respiratory tract interventional procedures.

Pleural fluid aspiration

Ultrasound is effective in diagnosing pleural fluid. Even small quantities can be visualized and aspirated for analysis.

Empyema drainage

Purulent fluid in the pleural cavity, usually due to infection from adjacent structures, can be drained directly by catheter insertion.

Bronchial wall stenting

In malignant narrowing of the bronchus, insertion of an expandable metal stent.

Embolization

Bronchial artery embolization in treatment of life-threatening haemoptysis, and embolization of pulmonary arterio-venous malformations.

Cardiovascular system

Angioplasty

Stenoses in the aorta, iliacs, femorals, peripheral vessels, carotids, coronary vessels, renals and virtually any other artery can be dilated by means of balloon inflation. Narrowed arterial segments and occlusions can also be

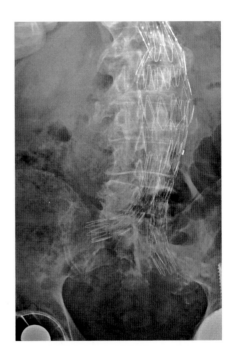

Figure 1.14 Aortic stent inserted via the femoral arteries for an aortic aneurysm.

treated by insertion of metallic stents. The superior vena cava can be stented to relieve malignant obstruction.

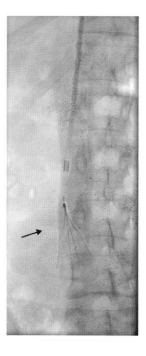

Figure 1.15 IVC filter insertion via the jugular vein (arrow).

Thrombolysis

Recent arterial thrombus can be lysed by positioning a catheter in the thrombus and infusing streptokinase or tissue plasminogen activator (TPA). Contraindications to this procedure include bleeding diatheses and recent cerebral infarction.

Embolization

The deliberate occlusion of arteries or veins for therapeutic purposes. Steel coils, detachable balloons or various other occluding agents are injected directly into the feeding vessels. Indications include arterial bleeding, arteriovenous fistulae and angiomatous malformations.

Vena cava filter insertion

A filter is introduced percutaneously through either the femoral or internal jugular vein and positioned in the inferior vena cava, just below the renal veins, thus preventing further embolization from the thrombus originating in pelvic or lower limb veins.

Aortic stenting (EVAR)

Used for the treatment of abdominal aortic aneurysms with insertion of the stent via the common femoral arteries.

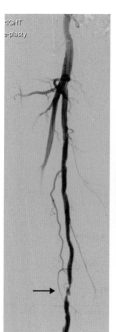
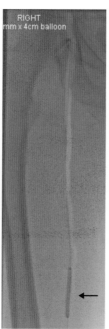
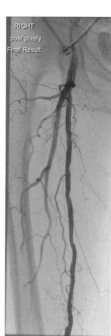

Figure 1.16 Arteriogram showing a femoral stenosis (arrow), subsequent balloon inflation in the stenosis (arrow), and following angioplasty showing a significant improvement in the stenosis.

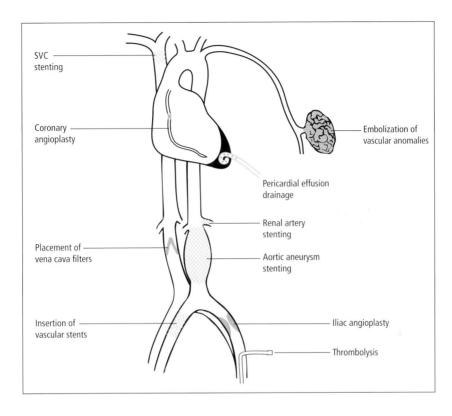

Figure 1.17 Cardiovascular system interventional procedures.

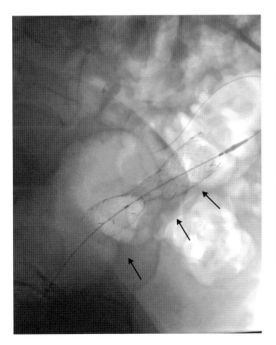

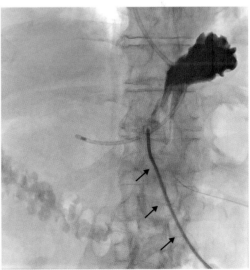

Figure 1.18 Colonic stent insertion (arrows) after a guidewire has been manoeuvred through the stricture and a stent deployed.

Figure 1.19 Percutaneous insertion of a gastrostomy (arrows). A nasogastric tube is in position.

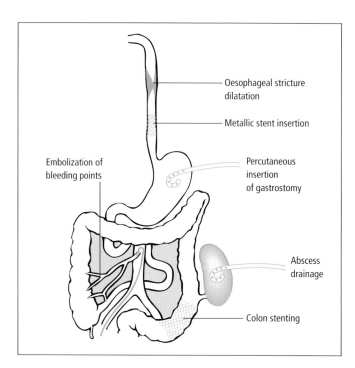

Figure 1.20 Gastrointestinal tract interventional procedures.

Oesophageal stricture dilatation

Metallic stent insertion

Embolization of bleeding points

Percutaneous insertion of gastrostomy

Abscess drainage

Colon stenting

Gastrointestinal tract

Oesophageal dilatation

A larger diameter balloon is used for dilatation of benign structures, postoperative anastomotic strictures (e.g. gastroenterostomy), achalasia and palliation of malignant strictures.

Oesophageal stent

A metallic self-expanding stent is inserted for palliation of malignant oesophageal strictures.

Colonic stent

Metal expandable stents can be inserted for palliation of malignant strictures.

Percutaneous gastrostomy

After gastric distension with air, a catheter is inserted directly through the anterior abdominal wall into the stomach.

Embolization

Angiography may localize the bleeding point in severe gastrointestinal haemorrhage. Control of haemorrhage may be possible by infusion of vasopressin or embolization.

Abscess drainage

Percutaneous drainage of subphrenic and pancreatic collections.

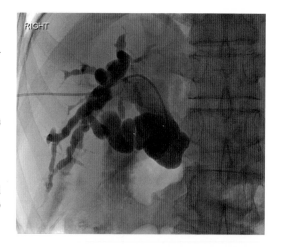

Figure 1.21 Cholangiogram showing complete biliary obstruction with marked dilatation of the intrahepatic bile ducts.

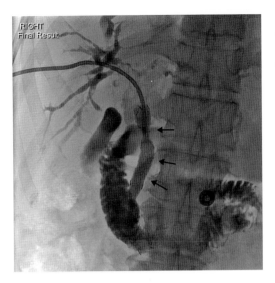

Figure 1.22 Biliary obstruction relieved by the insertion of a metal stent in the common bile duct (arrows).

Internal biliary drainage with endoprosthesis

A plastic or metal stent is positioned within the biliary stricture and free internal drainage achieved without the need for any external catheters. The procedure is preferably carried out by endoscopic retrograde cholangiopancreatography (ERCP), but if this fails, the stent can be inserted using a percutaneous approach.

Liver biopsy

Safer to perform with ultrasound control. Focal lesions can be biopsied for a histological diagnosis.

Biliary duct dilatation

Balloon dilatation of a benign biliary stricture.

Other

Liver/subphrenic abscess drainage and biliary stone removal.

Urinary tract
Renal angioplasty

Balloon dilatation of renal artery stenosis or insertion of metallic stents to alleviate the stenosis (treatment of hypertension or to preserve renal function).

Biliary tract
External biliary drainage

In biliary obstruction, a catheter is inserted percutaneously through the liver into the bile ducts.

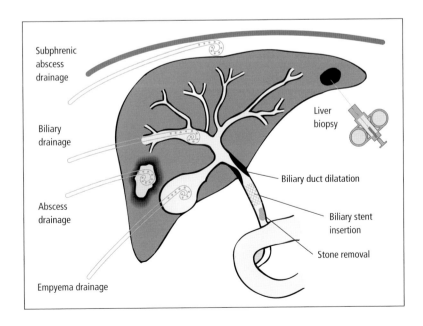

Figure 1.23 Biliary tract interventional procedures.

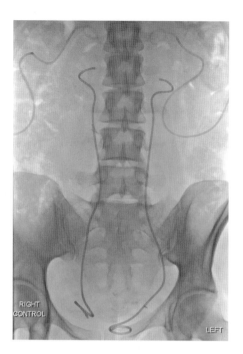

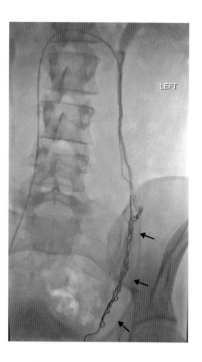

Figure 1.24 Percutaneous insertion of bilateral ureteric stents.

Figure 1.25 Venogram showing a catheter inserted via the right femoral and embolization coils deployed (arrows) for a left varicocele.

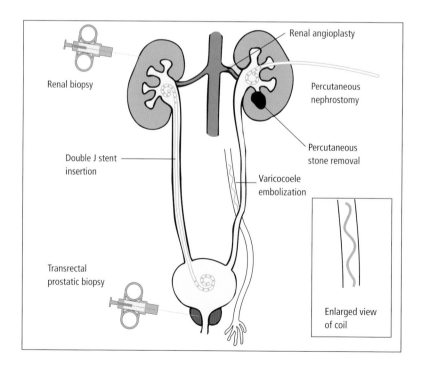

Renal angioplasty

Renal biopsy

Percutaneous nephrostomy

Double J stent insertion

Percutaneous stone removal

Varicocoele embolization

Transrectal prostatic biopsy

Enlarged view of coil

Figure 1.26 Interventional procedures of the urinary tract.

Percutaneous nephrostomy

To establish free drainage of urine when the kidney is obstructed, by insertion of a catheter into the pelvi-calyceal system.

Ureteric stent

A special catheter positioned, so one end lies in the renal pelvis and the other in the bladder, for the relief of obstruction. Introduction is either from the lower ureter after cystoscopy by an urologist or from above percutaneously under radiological control.

Percutaneous stone removal

Removal of a renal calculus, through a percutaneous track, from the posterior abdominal wall directly into the kidney.

Embolization

Useful in the treatment of bleeding A-V renal fistulae and to occlude the testicular vein in a varicocoele.

2

Respiratory tract

Respiratory tract investigations

Plain film images

The standard view used is the posteroanterior (PA) projection, with the patient's front against the digital plate and the X-ray beam directed through the back. Other projections include the following.

- Lateral: localizes an abnormality seen on the PA view.
- Anteroposterior (AP): used for ill patients; because of magnification, it is difficult to assess heart size on this projection.
- Supine: valuable in infants and ill patients; it is not possible to assess heart size on this view.
- Erect: detects gas under the diaphragm in a suspected abdominal viscus perforation.

The following projections are occasionally used.

- Oblique: useful to demonstrate pleural, chest wall and rib abnormalities.
- Apical: the patient stands erect and leans backwards to give a bone-free view of the lung apices.
- Expiratory: a pneumothorax becomes more prominent.

Computed tomography (CT)

CT is now an essential and indispensable modality in evaluating chest disease for the following reasons.

- It provides excellent detail for localizing and staging mediastinal masses and bronchial neoplasms.
- It assesses hilar areas to identify lymphadenopathy, and to differentiate from prominent pulmonary arteries.

- It accurately localizes pleural masses, plaques and fluid associated with asbestos exposure.
- It aids diagnosis of aortic aneurysm, aortic dissection or superior vena cava obstruction.
- It characterizes the nature of a lung opacity; identifies the presence of secondary deposits.
- It assists percutaneous lung biopsy.

High-resolution CT (HRCT), with thin slices of 1–2 mm thickness at 1–2 cm intervals, is used to assess parenchymal lung disease and to monitor progression, especially:

- interstitial lung disease such as pulmonary fibrosis;
- bronchiectasis showing dilated bronchi and cystic changes.

The following examples demonstrate the value of CT in the respiratory tract.

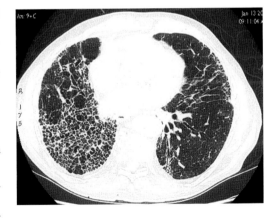

Figure 2.1 HRCT showing extensive lung fibrosis with some sparing of the left lung posteriorly.

Radiology: Lecture Notes, Fourth Edition. Pradip R. Patel.
© 2020 John Wiley & Sons Ltd. Published 2020 by John Wiley & Sons Ltd.
Companion website: www.wiley.com/go/patel/radiology

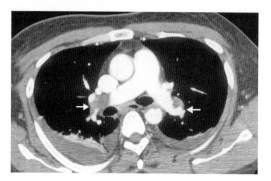

Figure 2.2 Contrast CT scan of the pulmonary arteries (CTPA): emboli in the right main pulmonary artery (→) and left lower lobe pulmonary artery (←) associated with pleural effusions.

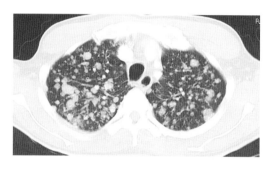

Figure 2.3 Widespread secondary deposits in the lungs.

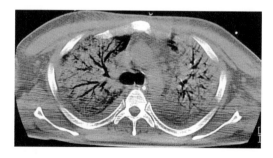

Figure 2.4 Extensive bilateral lung consolidation with an air bronchogram (air still present in the bronchi).

Ultrasound

Ultrasound examination of the chest determines the presence of pleural effusions and loculated fluid. It will accurately locate small quantities of fluid for aspiration. Biopsy of pleural lesions may be carried out using ultrasound guidance.

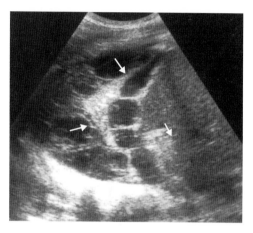

Figure 2.5 A loculated effusion on ultrasound with multiple septations (arrows). This will be difficult to aspirate to completion.

Lung biopsy

After infiltration with local anaesthetic, a needle is inserted directly into the mass to be biopsied, obtaining tissue samples. Biopsy should not be carried out if there is a suspicion of an arteriovenous malformation. Poor respiratory function is also a contraindication, as a pneumothorax following biopsy may seriously compromise the patient.

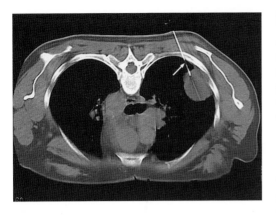

Figure 2.6 Lung biopsy under CT control. The needle (arrow) has been inserted through the posterior chest wall.

Isotopes

Combined perfusion scanning with technetium-99m-labelled macroaggregates of human albumin and ventilation scanning with inhaled radioactive gas or aerosol typically produces a perfusion defect and not a ventilation defect in pulmonary embolus.

Pulmonary angiography

This technique is now used only occasionally. The pulmonary artery is selectively catheterized, through either the jugular or femoral vein, and contrast injected to visualize the pulmonary arterial and venous circulation. This is an invasive procedure and should generally be reserved if CT pulmonary angiography is unsatisfactory.

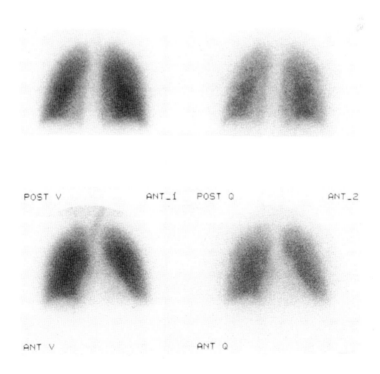

POST V   ANT_1   POST Q   ANT_2

ANT V   ANT Q

Figure 2.7 Normal ventilation (V) and perfusion (Q) scan.

PET scanning

PET uses radioactively labelled glucose to assess metabolic activity in tissues. It is a very useful imaging modality to see if lung nodules, pleural thickening or mediastinal lymph nodes contain tumour tissue. False positives can occur with inflammatory lesions and false negatives for some slow-growing tumours and metastases.

Magnetic resonance imaging (MRI)

The lungs are not well visualized with this technique, and is not in common use, but the principal indications are evaluation of mediastinal masses, aortic dissection and staging bronchial carcinoma, if vascular invasion is suspected.

Figure 2.8 (a) Normal chest X-ray; (b) normal lateral chest X-ray.

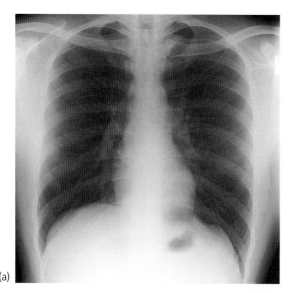

(a)

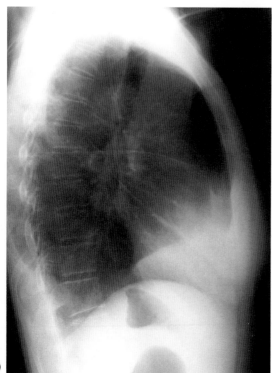

(b)

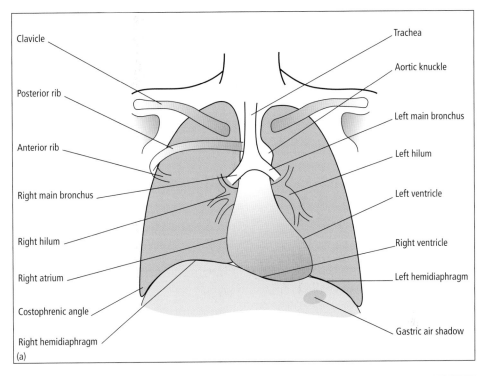

Clavicle

Posterior rib

Anterior rib

Right main bronchus

Right hilum

Right atrium

Costophrenic angle

Right hemidiaphragm

(a)

Trachea

Aortic knuckle

Left main bronchus

Left hilum

Left ventricle

Right ventricle

Left hemidiaphragm

Gastric air shadow

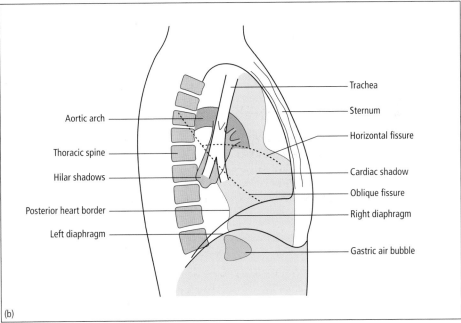

Aortic arch

Thoracic spine

Hilar shadows

Posterior heart border

Left diaphragm

(b)

Trachea

Sternum

Horizontal fissure

Cardiac shadow

Oblique fissure

Right diaphragm

Gastric air bubble

Figure 2.8 (Continued)

Normal chest

Some important radiological considerations

Hilar shadows

Predominantly due to pulmonary arteries: the left hilum is smaller and a little higher than the right.

Horizontal fissure

A white 'hair-line' shadow dividing the right upper and middle lobes and extending up to the right hilum; it is not always seen.

Cardiac shadow

The right atrium is seen just to the right of the thoracic spine. The inferior border is formed by the right ventricle and the left border by the left ventricle.

Diaphragm

The right leaf is usually higher than the left, though occasionally the converse may be true.

Trachea

Lies in the midline with bifurcation at the level of T6. It deviates slightly to the right at the level of the aortic knuckle.

Lung fields

The intrapulmonary arteries radiate from the pulmonary hila and taper towards the periphery contributing to the majority of the lung markings, with a smaller component from the pulmonary veins. The right lung is divided into three lobes: the upper, a small middle lobe and lower lobe. The left lung has two lobes, the upper (including the lingula) and lower.

Viewing a chest film

Inspect the film for adequate penetration (lower thoracic spine just visible), inspiration (diaphragms at level of fifth or sixth ribs anteriorly) and rotation (the spinous processes of the upper thoracic vertebrae lie midway between the medial ends of the clavicles).

Examine the chest X-ray systematically to ensure that all areas are covered; skeletal and soft tissues are best left to the end. Keep to a routine, but with practice it will be possible to spot the abnormalities and describe them first: lungs; hilar shadows; cardiac shadow; mediastinum; diaphragms; skeletal and soft tissues.

Lungs

Inspect both lungs, starting at the apices and working downwards. Compare the appearances of each zone with the other side. (The lungs can be divided approximately into three zones: the upper, middle and lower zones.) The only shadows normally visible, apart from the fissures, should be vascular in origin, so concentrate on searching for any areas of homogeneous shadowing or a mass lesion. It may be easier to describe an opacity within a zone and later determine the lung lobe.

Hilar shadows

A common site for lymphadenopathy and bronchial carcinoma: look for increased density and irregularity as well as enlargement of the hilar shadow.

Cardiac shadow

Note the size and shape. Specific chamber enlargement is often difficult to identify: pay attention to and comment on the overall size of the heart.

Mediastinum

Assess for mass lesions and also for mediastinal shift by position of the trachea and cardiac shadow.

Diaphragms

The costophrenic angles should be clear, sharp and deep. Blunting may indicate a pleural effusion or old pleural thickening. The upper surfaces should be clearly defined: poor definition often implies basal lung pathology. Flattening of the diaphragms suggests hyperinflation and chronic obstructive airways disease.

Skeletal and soft tissues

Look at the periphery of the film; ribs, for fractures or secondary deposits; appearances of the breast shadows and whether there has been a mastectomy; under diaphragms; shoulders; etc.

Principal types of lung shadowing

Normal appearances

The lungs appear translucent with only branches of the pulmonary arteries and veins visible. There is no other shadowing.

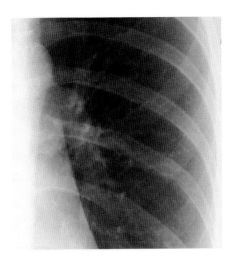

Figure 2.9 Normal lung fields.

Nodular shadowing

Nodular shadowing is due to small, discrete spherical opacities 1–5 mm in diameter. Causes include: miliary tuberculosis; pneumoconiosis; sarcoidosis; neoplastic: miliary carcinomatosis from thyroid, melanoma, etc.

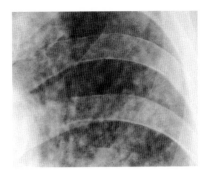

Figure 2.11 Nodular shadowing.

Reticular/interstitial shadowing

This is produced by thickening of the tissues around the alveoli, the lung interstitium, and visualized as a fine or coarse branching linear pattern. Typical conditions giving rise to this type of shadowing are lung fibrosis and pneumoconiosis.

Consolidation

Consolidation is due to replacement of air in the alveoli by fluid, or occasionally tissue, resulting in areas of confluent homogeneous shadowing. Patent bronchi and some small airways are often still visible as linear lucencies, when surrounded by fluid-filled alveoli; this sign is called an air bronchogram.

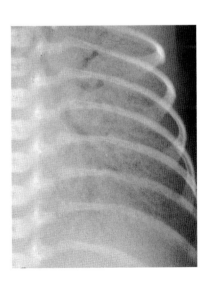

Figure 2.12 Consolidation showing an air bronchogram.

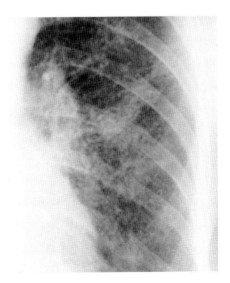

Figure 2.10 Interstitial lung shadowing.

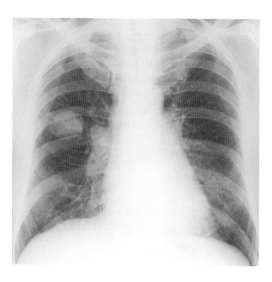

Figure 2.13 Bronchial carcinoma: solitary circular opacity in the right mid-zone ('coin lesion').

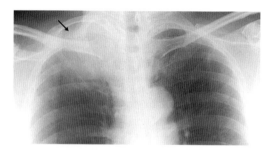

Figure 2.14 Pancoast's tumour at the right apex with rib destruction (arrow).

Bronchial carcinoma: peripheral

This is a common primary tumour, the main types being small cell lung cancer (SCLC) and non-small cell lung cancer (NSCLC), which have differing responses to therapy. The latter group includes adenocarcinoma, squamous cell and large cell carcinoma.

Presentation

Haemoptysis; respiratory symptoms such as cough and shortness of breath; weight loss; cerebral or lymph-node metastases; slowly resolving pneumonia; routine chest X-ray; paraneoplastic syndromes such as inappropriate antidiuretic hormone (ADH) secretion.

Radiological features

Bronchoscopy may be negative in peripheral lesions, as visualization is not possible distal to the segmental bronchi. The following features may be present on a plain chest film.

- Lobulated or spiculated mass, but sometimes with a smooth outline.
- Associated hilar gland enlargement, pleural effusion, areas of collapse or consolidation.
- Cavitation found in 15% with central air lucency, an air/fluid level and a wall of variable thickness. Squamous carcinomas frequently cavitate.
- Tumours at the lung apex (Pancoast's tumour) can invade the brachial plexus, resulting in shoulder and arm pain with wasting of the hand, or invasion of the sympathetic chain may give rise to Horner's syndrome.
  Further investigations include the following.
- *CT chest and upper abdomen.* Assesses spread and determines operability. This examination will establish whether there has been any metastatic spread into the mediastinal lymph nodes, chest wall, liver or adrenals. MRI is generally more accurate in defining mediastinal and vascular invasion.
- *PET or PET/CT* scan to determine metastatic spread.
- *Lung biopsy.* Either under fluoroscopy or CT control to obtain a sample for histology.

Differential diagnosis of a solitary lung mass

- Metastasis: sometimes single, most commonly from breast, kidney, colon and testicular tumours.
- Tuberculoma: often apical and may have areas of calcification.

- Benign neoplasms: bronchial adenoma (usually peri-hilar), hamartoma (most common benign tumour of the lung), rarely focal areas of pneumonia, hydatid cyst, haematoma or arteriovenous malformation.

> **Key point**
>
> Inspect the lungs carefully for a focal mass as lung cancer is a common neoplasm

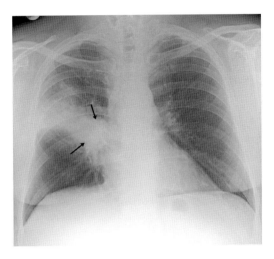

Figure 2.15 Central bronchial carcinoma (arrows) with peripheral consolidation.

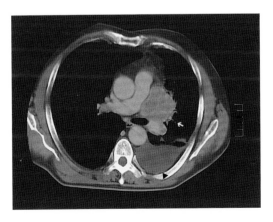

Figure 2.16 CT scan demonstrating the left hilar mass (arrow). There is no associated lymphadenopathy but a left pleural effusion is present (arrowhead).

Bronchial carcinoma: central

Central bronchial carcinoma arises from the major bronchi, causing a mass in the hilar region.

Presentation

As in peripheral carcinoma.

Radiological features

On a chest *X-ray*, the central mass causes the hilar shadow to enlarge, assume an increased density or an irregular outline. As the tumour increases in size, narrowing of the bronchial lumen may cause collapse of the distal lung and consolidation due to secondary infection. A large tumour often gives rise to complete collapse of a lung and may result in opacification of the entire hemithorax.

CT/CT PET/MRI aids identification of extent and spread of the tumour to:

- lymph nodes: mediastinal and hilar lymphadenopathy;
- oesophagus: direct invasion with dysphagia or fistula;
- pleura: pleural effusion;
- pericardium: pericardial effusion;
- bone: direct extension into sternum or ribs;
- superior vena cava: obstruction with venous engorgement.

Common sites of distant metastases are:

- brain;
- bone;
- adrenals;
- liver.

Lymphangitis carcinomatosa: dissemination of carcinoma through lymphatic channels of the lung, often unilateral, but may be bilateral.

Invasion of the tumour may also involve the phrenic nerve (elevation of the diaphragm) or laryngeal nerve (hoarseness).

Treatment

- Surgical resection: generally inoperable if direct chest wall invasion, mediastinal spread or distant metastases.
- Chemotherapy: especially for small cell carcinoma.
- Radiotherapy: inoperable tumours or when complications arise:
  - brain metastases;
  - spinal cord compression;
  - superior vena cava obstruction.

> **Key point**
>
> Central bronchial carcinoma is often difficult to identify and a smoker presenting with haemoptysis should be considered to have an underlying neoplasm

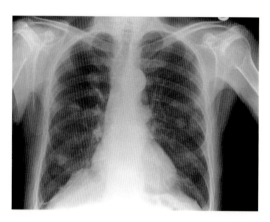

Figure 2.17 Focal lung secondary deposits.

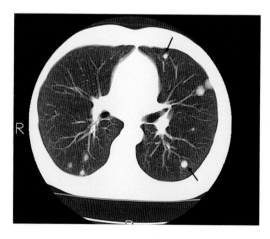

Figure 2.18 CT thorax showing multiple small metastases (arrows).

Pulmonary metastases

Metastatic disease to the lungs and rib cage is a common complication of primary neoplastic disease originating elsewhere, usually through the haematogenous route. Tumours of the breast, renal tract, testis, gastrointestinal tract, thyroid and bone are often the primary source.

Radiological features

Abnormalities can be seen on either plain films or CT. Metastatic disease to the chest may involve one or more of the following: lungs; pleura; lymph nodes; local invasion; bony skeleton.

Lungs

Virtually any malignancy may give secondary deposits in the lungs. Deposits usually appear as well-defined, multiple, round opacities of differing sizes in the lung fields. CT is particularly sensitive in detecting metastases not visible on a chest X-ray and helpful in monitoring response to chemotherapy. Opacities just a few millimetres across can be visualized easily. Cavitation is occasionally present, usually indicating metastases from squamous cell carcinoma.

Pleura

Pleural metastases are often from breast carcinoma, and may be visualized as mass lesions, though the most common manifestation is a pleural effusion, masking the underlying pathology.

Lymph nodes

CT is highly accurate in the detection of enlarged hilar and mediastinal lymph nodes (nodes less than 1 cm in the short axis diameter are less likely to be metastatic).

Lymphangitis carcinomatosa – secondary deposits in central lymph nodes may produce lymphatic congestion with a linear pulmonary pattern radiating outwards from the hilar glands, septal lines and pleural effusions.

Local invasion

Pericardium to give malignant pericardial effusion; superior vena cava compression or obstruction; phrenic nerve paralysis; Pancoast's tumour.

Skeletal system: ribs, thoracic spine, shoulder

Deposits may be lytic, e.g. from breast, sclerotic from prostate, or mixed.

> **Key point**
>
> Multiple lung lesions of varying size are invariably metastases

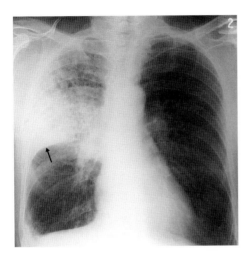

Figure 2.19 Right upper lobe pneumonia bounded inferiorly by the horizontal fissure (arrow). Blunting at the right costophrenic angle is due to a pleural effusion.

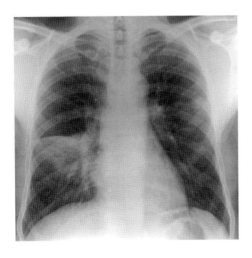

Figure 2.20 Right middle lobe pneumonia.

Pneumonia

Pneumonia, an inflammatory reaction in the lungs, occurs either as a primary infection of the lungs or secondary to bronchial obstruction.

Primary pneumonia

Inflammation arising in a normal lung.

Secondary pneumonia

Caused by:

- occluded bronchus from bronchial carcinoma or foreign body;
- aspiration from pharyngeal pouch, oesophageal obstruction;
- underlying lung pathology: bronchiectasis, cystic fibrosis.

Lobar pneumonia

Inflammatory changes confined to a lobe, classically due to *Streptococcus pneumoniae*.

Bronchopneumonia

Produces bilateral multifocal areas of consolidation.

Radiological features

It is generally not possible to diagnose the infecting agent from the type of shadowing. The affected part of the lung assumes an increased density with inflammatory exudate and fluid occupying the alveolar space. Air still remaining in the affected bronchi appears as linear lucencies (consolidation with air bronchogram). Consolidation may persist, often after the patient's symptoms have improved. CT is not required for primary pneumonia, but allows assessment of complications.

Types of pneumonia

- *Viral* pneumonia: most common pneumonia in children.
- *Streptococcal* pneumonia: commonest cause of bacterial pneumonia.

- *Mycoplasma* pneumonia (primary atypical pneumonia): commonest cause of non-bacterial pneumonia, often with slow resolution.
- *Staphylococcal* pneumonia: most frequent cause of bronchopneumonia and secondary invader in influenza.
- *Klebsiella* pneumonia: predominantly seen in elderly, debilitated patients.
- *Legionella* pneumonia: rapidly progressive, often in lower lobes with systemic involvement affecting liver and kidneys and other organs.
- *Pneumocystis carinii* pneumonia: typically in acquired immune deficiency syndrome (AIDS) or those immunosuppressed; diffuse perihilar changes progress to alveolar consolidation.
- Radiation pneumonia: pneumonic consolidation arising in the field of radiotherapy.

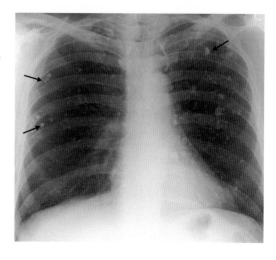

Figure 2.22 Old healed calcified tuberculous foci (arrows).

Key point

Pneumonic consolidation must be followed up to resolution to avoid missing an underlying bronchial carcinoma

Tuberculosis

Tuberculosis is a chronic infection caused by *Mycobacterium tuberculosis*, affecting mainly the respiratory tract, though it can involve any system in the body. The immigrant population, debilitated or immunosuppressed patients are all prone to the infection.

Radiological features

In *primary tuberculosis*, the following may be present on a chest X-ray.

- Area of peripheral pneumonic consolidation (Ghon focus) with enlarged hilar mediastinal glands (primary complex). This usually heals with calcification.
- Areas of consolidation, which may be small, lobar or more extensive throughout the lung fields.
  In *postprimary tuberculosis* or reactive tuberculosis, the following may be present.
- Patchy consolidation, especially in the upper lobes or apical segments of the lower lobes, often with cavitation.
- Pleural effusions, empyema or pleural thickening.
- Miliary tuberculosis: discrete 1–2 mm nodules distributed evenly throughout the lung fields due to haematogenous spread.
- Mediastinal or hilar lymphadenopathy is typically not a feature, except in AIDS patients.

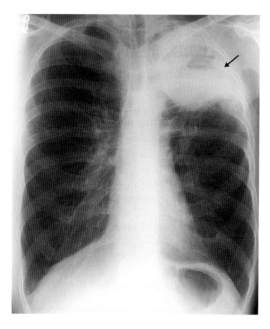

Figure 2.21 Cavitating consolidation in the left upper lobe: active tuberculosis (arrow).

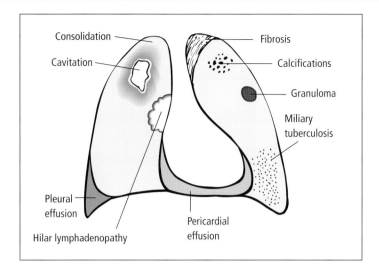

Figure 2.23 Manifestations of pulmonary tuberculosis.

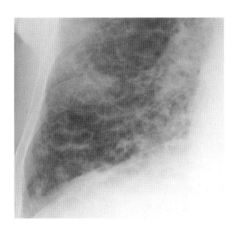

Figure 2.24 Cystic bronchiectasis: ring opacities at the right base.

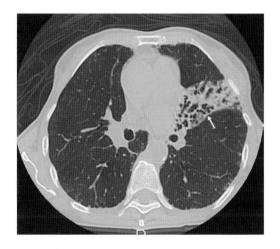

Figure 2.25 CT scan of thorax: bronchiectasis confined to the lingula (arrow).

As healing progresses, features that may be recognized are: fibrosis and volume loss; calcified foci; tuberculoma (a localized granuloma often containing calcification); pleural calcification.

> **Key point**
>
> Calcification in a lung lesion generally indicates a benign cause

Bronchiectasis

Bronchiectasis is defined as a condition in which there is an irreversible dilatation of the bronchi. The main aetiological factors appear to be obstruction leading to distal bronchial dilatation and infection causing permanent bronchial wall damage.

Presentation

Cough with purulent sputum; haemoptysis; recurrent chest infections.

Radiological features

The chest film may be entirely normal. Bronchiectasis is commonest at the lung bases and a chest X-ray may reveal the following features.

- *Cylindrical bronchiectasis*: dilated bronchi may be visible as parallel lines (representing the bronchial walls) radiating from the hilum towards the diaphragm.
- *Cystic bronchiectasis*: terminal dilatation may be visualized as cystic or ring shadows, sometimes with fluid levels.
- Pneumonic consolidation.
- Fibrotic changes.

HRCT unequivocally demonstrates bronchial dilatation and thickened bronchial walls. It can also define which lobes are affected, especially important to identify if surgery is needed. On CT, the following additional features may be observed:

- bronchi visible peripherally;
- bronchus larger in diameter than the adjacent pulmonary artery branch.

Complications

Empyema; cerebral abscess; amyloid.

Causes

- Childhood infections: following measles and whooping cough complicated by pneumonia.
- Aspergillosis: hypersensitivity reaction in the bronchial walls in asthmatics resulting in bronchiectasis which affects proximal airways.
- Bronchial obstruction: foreign body, neoplasm or tuberculosis.
- Cystic fibrosis: viscid sputum leading to bronchial obstruction and bronchiectasis.
- Congenital: Kartagener's syndrome (dextrocardia, sinusitis and bronchiectasis).

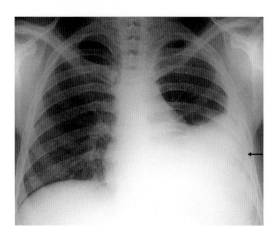

Figure 2.26 Large left pleural effusion (arrow).

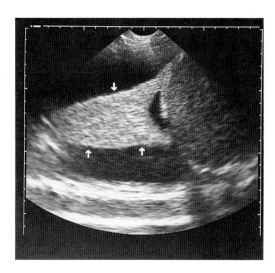

Figure 2.27 Ultrasound showing the effusion (black) surrounding the retracted lung (arrows).

Pleural effusion

Pleural effusion, a fluid collection in the space between the parietal and visceral layers of the pleura, usually contains serous fluid, but may have differing contents.

Haemothorax: Blood, usually following trauma.

Empyema: Purulent fluid from extension of pneumonia or lung abscess.

Chylothorax: Chyle from thoracic duct rupture or from malignant invasion.

Hydropneumothorax: Fluid and air.

> **Key point**
>
> The minimum fluid volume that can be visualized on a chest film is 200–300 ml; this will blunt the costophrenic angle

Radiological investigations

Chest film; ultrasound; CT.

Radiological appearances

Pleural fluid, in the erect position, gravitates to the lowermost part of the thorax with the following features on a chest X-ray:

- homogeneous opacification, similar density as the cardiac shadow;
- loss of the diaphragm outline;
- no visible pulmonary or bronchial markings;
- concave upper border with the highest level in the axilla.

As the fluid collection grows in size, the underlying lung decreases in volume and retracts towards the hilum. Initially the fluid accumulates in the posterior, then the lateral costophrenic space. With larger effusions, there is a mediastinal shift to the opposite side.

Subpulmonary effusion

Caused by fluid accumulating between the diaphragm and the inferior part of the lung. The upper margin of the shadow of the fluid runs parallel to the diaphragm and on the PA chest film mimics a high diaphragm.

Loculated effusion

Fluid can loculate in the fissures or against the chest wall, and this is occasionally seen in cardiac failure.

- Ultrasound is a highly sensitive examination in detecting pleural fluid.
- CT may also demonstrate pleural effusions and visualize underlying abnormalities.

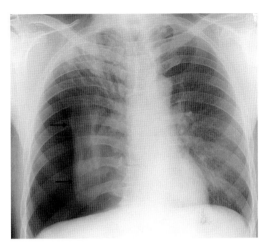

Figure 2.28 Right pneumothorax: there are no visible markings beyond the lung edge (arrows).

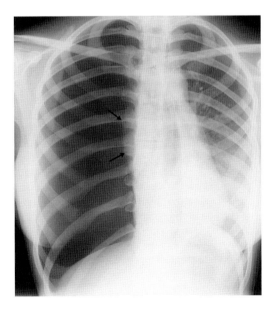

Figure 2.29 Tension pneumothorax with complete collapse of the right lung (arrows) and mediastinal shift to the left.

Pneumothorax

A pneumothorax occurs when air enters the pleural cavity via a tear in either the parietal or visceral pleura; the lung subsequently relaxes and retracts to a varying extent towards the hilum.

Radiological features

Pneumothorax is best demonstrated on an under-penetrated chest film. The following may be seen.

- Lung edge: a thin white line of the lung margin, the visceral pleura.
- Absent lung markings between the lung edge and chest wall.
- Mediastinal shift: when a tension pneumothorax develops.

Causes

- Iatrogenic (one of the commonest causes): following lung biopsy, chest aspiration, thoracic surgery and central line insertion.
- Spontaneous: most common in tall, thin, young males; usually due to rupture of a small pleural bleb.
- Trauma: stab wounds, rib fractures. Surgical emphysema is commonly associated with air tracking along the muscle planes of the chest wall.
- Pre-existing lung disease: increased incidence of pneumothorax with underlying lung disease such as emphysema, cystic fibrosis or interstitial lung disease.

Complications

- Tension pneumothorax: a tear in the visceral pleura may act as a ball valve allowing air to enter the pleural cavity during each inspiration and none to escape during expiration. Positive pressure builds up, resulting in a dramatic shift of the mediastinum away from the side of the pneumothorax. This is a medical emergency, as death can rapidly ensue from respiratory distress and diminished cardiac output.
- Hydropneumothorax: fluid in a pneumothorax.

Treatment

Generally, a small pneumothorax with less than 20% collapse of the lung requires no treatment. Pleural air will reabsorb with subsequent lung expansion. Larger pneumothoraces can be treated by aspiration or insertion of a chest drain with an underwater seal. Follow-up films are required to ensure complete resolution of the pneumothorax.

> **Key point**
>
> As air rises in an upright patient, a pneumothorax is most commonly seen at the apex

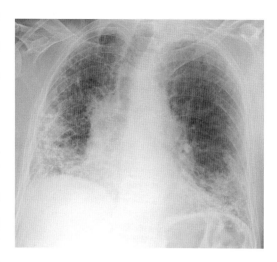

Figure 2.30 Extensive lung fibrosis.

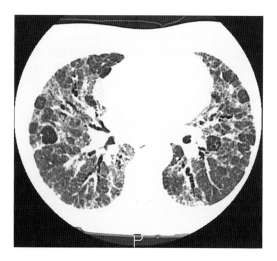

Figure 2.31 CT thorax: fibrosing alveolitis with coarse linear fibrotic strands.

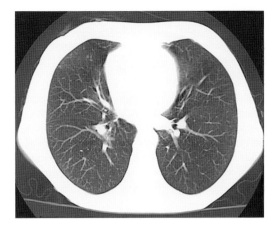

Figure 2.32 Normal CT thorax at the same level.

Idiopathic pulmonary fibrosis

Idiopathic pulmonary fibrosis is a disease of unknown aetiology characterized by diffuse interstitial lung fibrosis, and may be a response to stimuli such as cigarette smoke, pollutants, drugs or infection. It is more common in males, and in the 40–70 age group. Prognosis is poor, with greater than 50% mortality over five years.

Presentation

Progressive dyspnoea; cough; finger clubbing.

Radiological features

In early disease, the chest X-ray may be normal, but as fibrosis progresses, the following features may exist.

- Fine nodular and streaky linear shadowing (reticulonodular pattern) starting at the bases but may involve all the lung fields.
- Honeycomb pattern in severe disease, with small cystic spaces and coarse reticulonodular shadowing.
- Reduction in lung volume.
- Poor definition of the cardiac outline due to adjacent lung fibrosis.
- Dilatation of pulmonary arteries with right ventricular enlargement and pulmonary hypertension.

HRCT sections define lung parenchymal changes earlier and the examination is more precise than a chest X-ray, identifying reticular opacities and honeycombing. CT is effective in monitoring progress of the disease.

Causes of lung fibrosis

- Sarcoidosis.
- Cystic fibrosis.
- Pneumoconiosis.
- Rheumatoid lung.
- Systemic sclerosis.
- Drugs: nitrofurantoin, cyclophosphamide.

Complications

- Pneumothorax.
- Cor pulmonale.

Treatment

- Steroids.
- Immunosuppressive therapy.

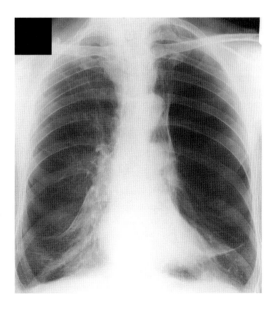

Figure 2.33 Emphysema: over-inflation of the lungs, flattened diaphragms, bullae and a small cardiac shadow.

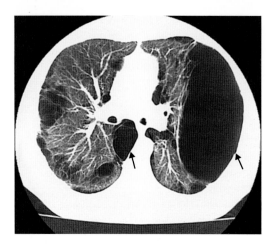

Figure 2.34 CT thorax: multiple destructive areas resulting in bullae of varying sizes (arrows).

Emphysema

Emphysema is a condition in which there is an increase in the size of the air spaces, with dilatation and destruction of lung tissue distal to the terminal bronchiole. Cigarette smokers and coal miners have a higher incidence and rarely there may be an association with α_1-antitrypsin deficiency (in which emphysema predominantly affects the lower lobes).

Radiological features

The chest X-ray may be entirely normal despite severe debility of the patient. In advanced emphysema, the following may be found.

Hyperinflation of the chest

- Low, flat diaphragms with limited excursion in inspiration and expiration.
- Increase in the AP diameter of the chest with an expansion in the retrosternal clear space (barrel chest).
- Thin, long and narrow appearance to the heart shadow, likely to be from over-inflation and low diaphragms, rather than an actual change in heart size.

Vascular changes

- The lungs are generally unevenly affected with an abnormal distribution of pulmonary vasculature; blood vessels are attenuated, with loss of the normal smooth gradation of vessels from the hilum to the periphery.

- Pulmonary hypertension leading to cor pulmonale. The proximal pulmonary arteries progressively enlarge and right-heart failure develops.

Bullae

Cyst-like spaces often develop from rupture of distended alveoli. On a chest film they are seen as translucent areas, with their walls shown as thin curvilinear hairline shadows. They vary in size from a few centimetres in diameter to occupying a large part of the hemithorax, displacing and compressing adjacent normal lung.

Terminology

The term 'emphysema' is also used in the following.

- *Mediastinal emphysema*: air within tissue planes of the mediastinum.
- *Surgical emphysema*: air tracking along the soft tissue planes; in the chest, this may be found after thoracic surgery or a pneumothorax.
- *Obstructive emphysema*: a bronchus partially occluded by a mass or foreign body causing a ball valve obstruction.

> **Key point**
>
> A large bulla in severe bullous emphysema may be mistaken for a pneumothorax

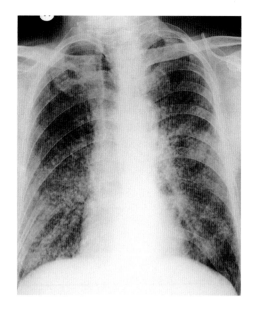

Figure 2.35 Coal worker's pneumoconiosis: coarse nodular shadowing.

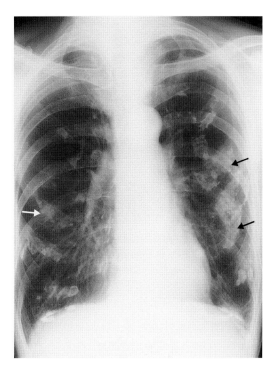

Figure 2.36 Calcified pleural plaques in asbestos exposure (arrows).

Pneumoconiosis

Pneumoconiosis is a condition caused by the inhalation of dust into the lungs. A history of dust exposure is present.

Radiological appearances

Appearances depend on whether the dust is active or inactive.

Active dust: Silica and coal dust are potent producers of diffuse lung fibrosis, although in the early stages small lung nodules are a characteristic feature.

Inactive dust: Iron oxide, calcium compounds and barium produce a fine nodular pattern, due to deposits of dust particles.

Organic dust: Exposure can also cause lung fibrosis, examples include the following.

- Bird-fancier's lung: pigeon and budgerigar excreta.
- Farmer's lung: mouldy hay.
- Bagassosis: sugar-cane dust.

Complications

- Progressive massive fibrosis.
- Caplan's syndrome.
- Emphysema.
- Cor pulmonale.

Asbestos exposure

Radiological appearances

With previous exposure to asbestos, the following may be seen on a chest X-ray.

- Focal pleural plaques: often the earliest finding, seen lying adjacent to ribs.
- Calcified pleural plaques: bilateral diaphragmatic calcifications are very suggestive of previous asbestos contact.
- Diffuse pleural thickening.
- Pleural effusions: often bilateral.
- Pulmonary fibrosis, especially basal, though the whole lung may be involved leading to cor pulmonale. Reticular shadowing commences at the bases and may obscure the sharp outline of the heart border.
- Malignant disease. There is a much higher incidence of:
  - mesothelioma (chest and peritoneal);
  - bronchial carcinoma, laryngeal carcinoma.

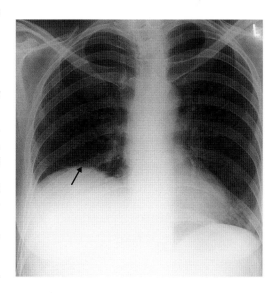

Figure 2.37 Elevated right diaphragm (arrow).

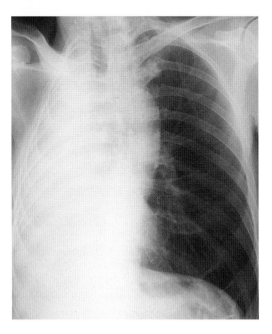

Figure 2.38 Complete opacification of the right hemithorax: collapse of the right lung with significant mediastinal shift to the right (note the position of the trachea and cardiac shadow).

Elevated diaphragm

The diaphragm consists of a thin sheet of muscle with a smooth upward convexity, the right usually lying in a higher position than the left. On a chest film, the inferior surface of the diaphragm is not visualized as it blends with the surfaces of the liver and spleen.

Causes of a unilateral elevated diaphragm

- Above diaphragm: phrenic nerve palsy; infiltration from bronchial carcinoma or mediastinal tumour.
- Diaphragm: eventration, more common on the left and results from deficiency or atrophy of muscle.
- Below diaphragm: right diaphragm elevation; liver or subphrenic abscess; liver secondary deposits.

Causes of bilateral elevated diaphragms

- Obesity.
- Hepatosplenomegaly.
- Within the abdomen: ascites, pregnancy, abdominal masses.

Opaque hemithorax

Complete opacification of a hemithorax is encountered in the following conditions. (Mediastinal shift is assessed by the position of the trachea and the heart.)

With mediastinal shift away from opaque hemithorax

Pleural effusion; large pleural effusions may occupy the whole of the hemithorax.

With mediastinum central

Consolidation; in severe pneumonia, consolidation may render the whole lung opaque.

With mediastinal shift towards opaque hemithorax

- Lung collapse: most commonly occurs from total occlusion of a main bronchus either by a central bronchial carcinoma or a postoperative mucus plug. The lung collapses and is devoid of air, hence the appearance of a dense hemithorax.
- Post pneumonectomy: after resection of a lung, the empty hemithorax fills with fluid. Gradual reabsorption with a fibrotic reaction eventually results in opacification with a significant mediastinal shift towards the pneumonectomy.

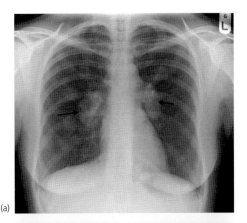

(a)

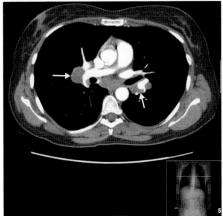

(b)

Figure 2.39 (a) Bilateral hilar lymphadenopathy (arrows); (b) contrast-enhanced CT showing hilar lymphadenopathy (arrows).

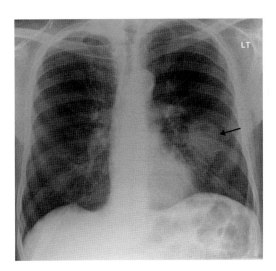

Figure 2.40 Lung abscess (arrow).

Hilar lymphadenopathy

Hilar lymphadenopathy may cause enlargement of the hilar shadows, the lymph nodes appearing as well-defined, lobulated masses. Nodal enlargement has to be differentiated from hilar vascular prominence (as in pulmonary hypertension). Difficulty may be encountered in distinguishing between them on chest radiography, though CT with contrast or MRI accurately identifies the abnormality.

Causes of bilateral hilar gland enlargement

- Sarcoidosis: commonest cause, usually resolving spontaneously.
- Lymphoma: mediastinal glands are more frequently involved than hilar.
- Tuberculosis: enlargement is usually asymmetrical and often associated with mediastinal glandular involvement.
- Metastases.

Causes of unilateral hilar gland enlargement

- Bronchial carcinoma.
- Lymphoma.
- Tuberculosis.

> **Key point**
>
> Asymptomatic bilateral hilar lymphadenopathy is often due to sarcoidosis

Lung abscess

A lung abscess is a localized, necrotic, cavitating lesion due to a pyogenic infection. Secondary abscess formation may occur from aspiration under anaesthesia, inhalation of vomit or foreign body, oesophageal disease such as achalasia or carcinoma of the oesophagus, or septic material aspiration from upper airway passages.

Radiological features

Abscess formation may initially start as an area of pneumonic consolidation (especially *Staphylococcus aureus* or *Klebsiella pneumoniae*) with subsequent development of cavitation. A fluid level is often noted in the abscess.

Differential diagnosis of a cavitating lesion

- Carcinoma: primary bronchial carcinoma is the commonest cause; solitary cavitating secondary deposit. A benign cavity has a central cavity and a regular wall, whereas a malignant one has an eccentric cavity with an irregular wall.
- Tuberculosis.
- Cavitating pulmonary infarct, haematoma or infected bulla (rare).

Key point

With a cavitating lesion, always exclude a cavitating bronchial carcinoma

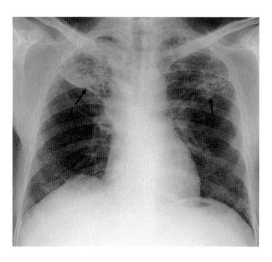

Figure 2.41 Upper zone fibrosis from tuberculosis (arrows).

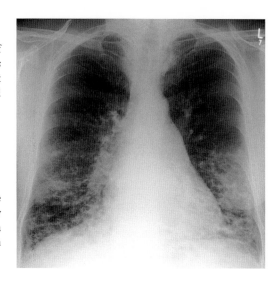

Figure 2.42 Lower zone fibrosis due to bronchiectasis.

Upper zone fibrosis

Fibrosis may affect predominantly the apices and upper zones, with sparing of the lower zones in the following conditions.

- Tuberculosis: associated with calcified areas and pleural thickening.
- Sarcoidosis: hilar lymphadenopathy may also be present.
- Radiotherapy: usually following treatment for carcinoma of the breast.
- Ankylosing spondylitis: fibrosis usually occurs when the spinal disease is severe.
- Chronic extrinsic allergic alveolitis: hypersensitivity reaction to inhalation of specific antigens, e.g. from pigeons and budgerigars; the chest X-ray is often normal but may show patchy consolidation in the acute stages, but in chronic disease, fibrotic shadowing is predominantly in the upper zones.

Lower zone fibrosis

Fibrosis in the lower zones may obscure the heart border and produce a 'shaggy heart' appearance. Fibrosis predominantly affects the lower zones in:

- bronchiectasis or long-standing infection;
- cryptogenic fibrosing alveolitis;
- rheumatoid arthritis;
- radiotherapy: usually following treatment for carcinoma of the breast;
- asbestos exposure;
- scleroderma: an autoimmune disease with fibrosis of interstitial lung tissue, predominantly basal but may involve the whole lung. The disease commonly affects the joints, skin, gut and respiratory tract.

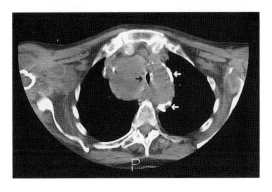

Figure 2.44 CT upper thorax: retrosternal thyroid causing tracheal narrowing (→). Note calcified areas in the mass (←).

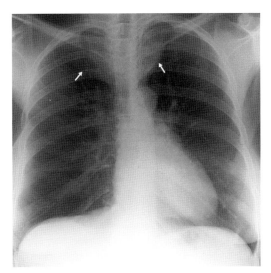

Figure 2.43 Widening of the upper mediastinum from a retrosternal thyroid (arrows).

Mediastinal mass

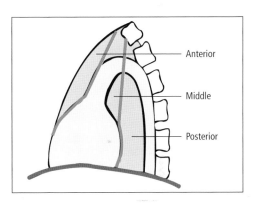

Figure 2.45 Mediastinal compartments.

The mediastinum is that part of the chest bounded by the sternum at the front, thoracic spine at the back and laterally by the medial surfaces of visceral pleura. It can be divided into:

- anterior mediastinum: anterior to the pericardium;
- middle mediastinum: the heart, aortic root and pulmonary vessels;

- posterior mediastinum: behind the posterior pericardial surface.

Although the mediastinum is categorized into compartments, masses may freely cross from one part to another.

Radiological features

Usually, a mediastinal mass is suspected on a plain chest film; a lateral film may be helpful; further evaluation is carried out by CT/MRI for anatomical localization. The presence of cystic lesions, calcification, fat and vascular structures are all more accurately assessed than by plain films.

Anterior mediastinal masses (three Ts – thyroid, thymus and teratodermoids)

- Retrosternal thyroid: the mass is well defined and may be lobulated. Extension into the mediastinum is to a varying degree up to the carina.
- Thymic tumours: these may be benign or malignant and frequently associated with myasthenia gravis.
- Teratodermoids: these tumours are usually benign but have a malignant potential. Occasionally fat, rim calcification, bone fragments and teeth may be identified.

Middle mediastinal masses

- Lymphadenopathy: lymphoma, metastases, sarcoid or tuberculosis.

Posterior mediastinal masses

- Neurogenic tumours arising from intercostal nerves and sympathetic chain.
- Neurofibromas (nerve sheath tumours).
- Ganglioneuroma (sympathetic nerve cell tumours).

> **Key point**
>
> 90% of posterior mediastinal masses are of neurogenic origin

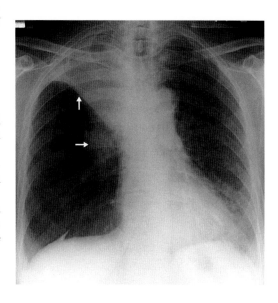

Figure 2.46 Right upper lobe collapse (↑) due to a mass at the right hilum (→).

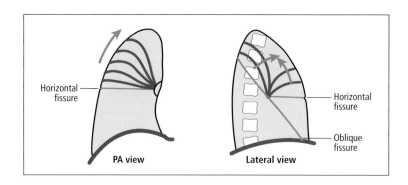

Figure 2.47 Movement of the fissures in right upper lobe collapse.

Right upper lobe collapse

The right upper lobe collapses with movement of the horizontal fissure upwards, pivoting at the hilum in both the PA and lateral projections. The collapsed lobe assumes an increased density at the right apex, its lower border being sharply defined by the horizontal fissure. The hilum may be elevated.

Right middle lobe collapse

The middle lobe is relatively small. On the PA view, middle lobe collapse produces only minor changes, with some increased density lateral to the right cardiac border with blurring of the cardiac outline (silhouette sign). It is most accurately evaluated using the lateral projection, where the collapsed lobe is seen as a triangular opacity projected over the cardiac shadow.

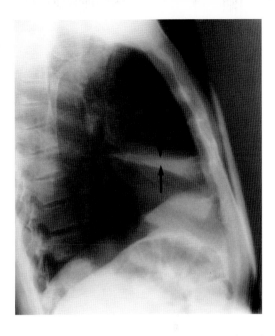

Figure 2.49 Lateral view showing the collapse projected over the cardiac shadow (arrows).

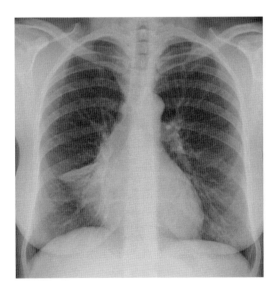

Figure 2.48 Right middle lobe collapse. PA view. Note the loss of right heart border.

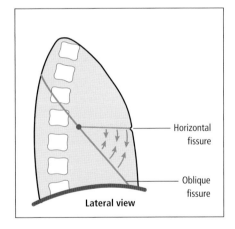

Figure 2.50 Movement of fissures in right middle lobe collapse.

Left upper lobe collapse

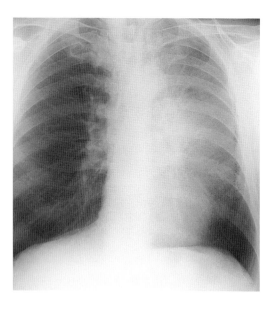

Figure 2.51 Left upper lobe collapse with hazy ill-defined shadowing in the left upper and mid-zone.

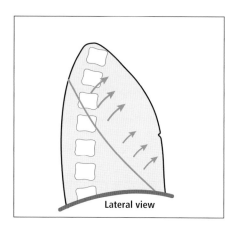

Figure 2.53 The oblique fissure moves forwards in left upper lobe collapse.

The lobe collapses in a different fashion to the right upper lobe. Movement of the oblique fissure is forwards and the collapsed lobe lies anteriorly against the chest wall, giving rise to a hazy, ill-defined opacity in the upper and mid-zones on the PA projection.

Right/left lower lobe collapse

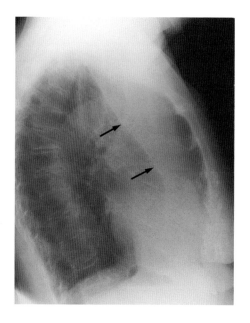

Figure 2.52 Lateral view shows the lobe collapse anteriorly (arrows).

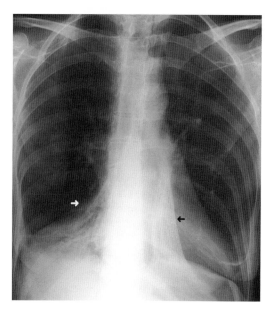

Figure 2.54 Bilateral lower lobe collapse (arrows), the left more clearly defined.

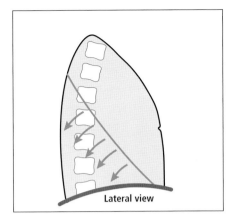

Lateral view

Figure 2.55 The oblique fissure moves backwards in lower lobe collapse.

The lower lobes collapse medially and posteriorly. The oblique fissure moves backwards maintaining the same slope. On the PA film, left lower lobe collapse is seen as a triangular area projected through the cardiac shadow.

3

Cardiovascular system

Cardiovascular investigations

Plain films

Evaluate heart size and chamber enlargement. On a standard PA chest projection, the ratio of the cardiac diameter to that of the maximum internal diameter of the chest should be no greater than 50% on a full inspiratory film. Expiratory films may falsely give the impression of cardiomegaly and pulmonary congestion. Supine films may also give a similar appearance.

Ultrasound

Echocardiography and Doppler examination reveal anatomical abnormalities as well as flow disturbances and assist in the study of incompetent and stenotic valves and ventricular function; aortic arch aneurysms, dissecting aneurysms, cardiomyopathy and pericardial effusions can also be diagnosed using echocardiography.

Ultrasound is a valuable technique of demonstrating the carotid arteries and any associated stenoses.

Isotope scanning

Technetium-99m pyrophosphate accumulates in damaged myocardium, whereas thallium-201 produces a deficient uptake in territories supplied by occluded or narrowed arteries. Thallium is most commonly used as a screening technique in patients with suspected coronary artery disease.

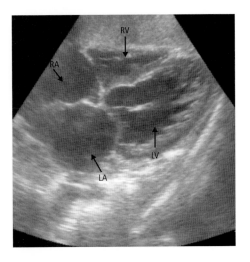

Figure 3.1 Ultrasound of the heart showing all four chambers: right atrium, right ventricle, left atrium and left ventricle (arrows).

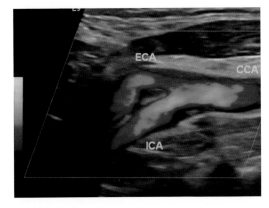

Figure 3.2 Normal Doppler scan showing the Carotid Bifurcation common carotid artery (CCA) bifurcating into the external carotid artery (ECA) and the internal carotid artery (ICA).

Radiology: Lecture Notes, Fourth Edition. Pradip R. Patel.
© 2020 John Wiley & Sons Ltd. Published 2020 by John Wiley & Sons Ltd.
Companion website: www.wiley.com/go/patel/radiology

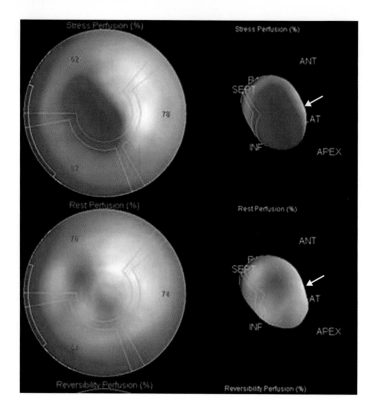

Figure 3.3 Isotope scan showing reduced cardiac perfusion during exercise (arrow, bottom scan) and normal perfusion at rest (arrow, top scan) showing reversible cardiac ischaemia.

Computed tomography (CT)

Relevant applications include the further evaluation and diagnosis of dissecting thoracic aneurysms, pericardial effusions and myocardial tumours. CT can calculate the total calcium deposition in the coronary arteries giving a predictive value of coronary artery disease. The latest generation of fast scanners provides accurate visualization of the coronary arteries.

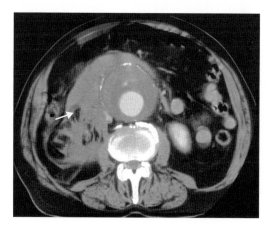

Figure 3.4 CT abdomen. Leaking abdominal 67 Insert aortic aneurysm with periaortic haematoma (arrow).

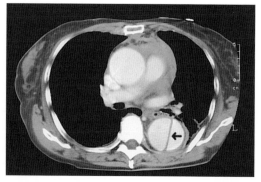

Figure 3.5 Dissection of the descending aorta. Note the intimal flap in the contrast-filled aorta (arrow) and blood in the mediastinum.

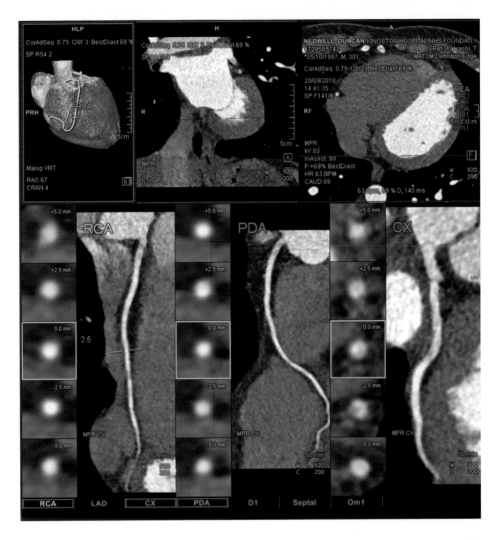

Figure 3.6 CT coronary angiogram shows a non-invasive method of clearly demonstrating the coronary arteries.

Magnetic resonance imaging (MRI)

MRI can be gated to the cardiac cycle to reduce motion artefact. It examines the heart in any plane and is of value in many clinical situations, including pericardial effusions, hypertrophic cardiomyopathy, and congenital and valvular heart disease. Magnetic resonance angiography (MRA) has the capability of providing a non-invasive method of imaging many vascular abnormalities, such as aneurysm, dissection, stenoses, occlusions and congenital anomalies.

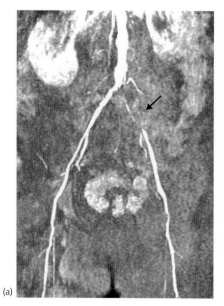

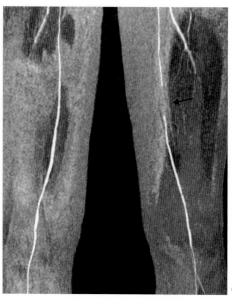

(a)

(b)

Figure 3.7 (a) MRI showing a left iliac artery occlusion (arrow). (b) MRI showing a left femoral artery occlusion (arrow).

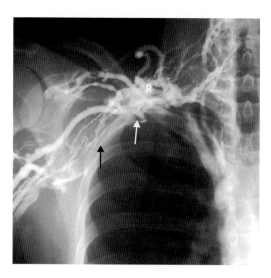

Figure 3.8 Right upper limb venography showing thrombus in the axillary and subclavian veins (arrows) with a large collateral circulation.

Venography

The venous system can be studied by proximal contrast injection. The most common indications are injection into:

- a foot vein to look at the lower limb venous system;
- antecubital vein to assess the axillary and subclavian vein and the superior vena cava (SVC);
- femoral vein to study the inferior vena cava (IVC).

Arteriography

Vascular access is usually obtained using a percutaneous approach via the femoral artery. Any major vessel or blood supply to an organ can be studied by selective arterial cannulation with contrast injection. Radial, brachial, axillary or popliteal arteries can also be punctured percutaneously, if femoral artery access is unsuitable. Anatomical detail is excellent; haematoma, haemorrhage and arterial thrombus are recognized rare local complications.

Coronary angiography is a commonly performed examination. In this study, contrast is initially injected into the left ventricle to evaluate function, and subsequently into the left and right main coronary arteries to detect the extent of any stenoses; angioplasty and stent insertion may be carried out on suitable stenoses.

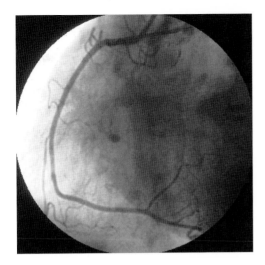

Figure 3.9 Normal right coronary angiogram.

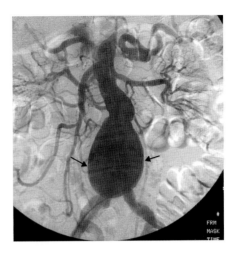

Figure 3.12 Aortogram: lower abdominal aortic aneurysm (arrows).

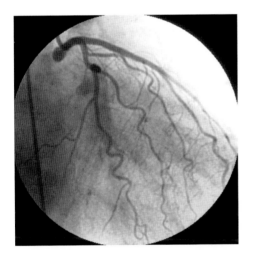

Figure 3.10 Normal left coronary angiogram.

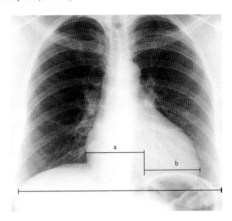

Figure 3.13 Cardiomegaly: the heart size is measured by comparing the cardiac diameter (a + b) to the maximum internal diameter of the chest.

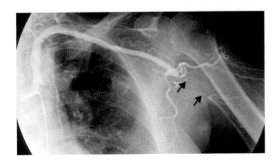

Figure 3.11 Left subclavian angiogram: short occlusion of the axillary artery (arrows).

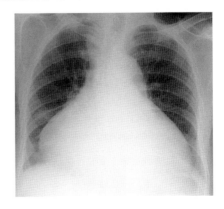

Figure 3.14 Pericardial effusion: large globular-shaped cardiac shadow with clear lung fields.

Cardiomegaly

On a standard PA chest, the heart size can be expressed as the cardiothoracic ratio. Generally, a ratio of over 50% of the heart size to the maximum internal diameter of the chest indicates cardiac enlargement. This measurement is only an approximate guide, and useful for serial measurement. Echocardiography is more accurate in the assessment of specific chamber and cardiac enlargement but a plain chest film may show the following.

- Left atrium: the only chamber enlargement reliably diagnosed; it may feature:
  - double contour to the right heart border;
  - splaying of the carina with upward displacement of the left main bronchus;
  - posterior bulging of the chamber on a lateral chest X-ray.
- Right atrium: prominence of the right heart border.
- Right ventricle: upward displacement of the cardiac apex with anterior enlargement of the heart border on a lateral projection.
- Left ventricle: increased convexity of left heart border.

> **Key point**
>
> Cardiac size assessment is difficult on AP and supine films

Pericardial effusion

A pericardial effusion is a collection of fluid in the pericardial sac, the fluid being either serous, blood or lymphatic in origin.

Radiological features

- *Chest film*: illustrates a symmetrically enlarged and globular cardiac shadow only when there is a significant effusion (>250 ml). Pericardial effusion should be suspected if there has been a rapid serial increase in the cardiac shadow, with normal pulmonary vasculature.
- *Echocardiography*: the investigation of choice. Effusions are visible as echo-free areas surrounding the heart.
- CT: may also identify the aetiology, e.g. mediastinal malignancy.
- MRI: accurate for diagnosis and also images the chest and mediastinum.

Causes

Infective (viral, bacterial, tuberculous); uraemia; postmyocardial infarction (Dressler's syndrome); myxoedema; malignancy: bronchial and mediastinal tumours with pericardial invasion; collagen vascular diseases (systemic lupus erythematosus (SLE), rheumatoid arthritis).

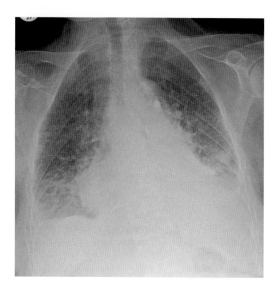

Figure 3.15 Congestive cardiac failure with interstitial pulmonary oedema.

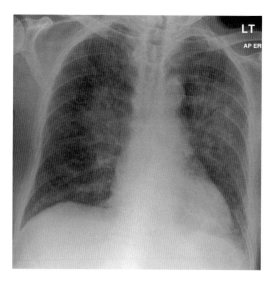

Figure 3.16 Alveolar pulmonary oedema; fluid accumulating predominantly in the perihilar region.

Cardiac failure

Cardiac failure is said to be present when tissue demands cannot be adequately supplied by the heart. It is usually due to low output from ischaemic heart disease but, paradoxically, may rarely result from high output as a consequence of excessive tissue needs in conditions such as thyrotoxicosis or Paget's disease.

Radiological features

On a chest X-ray, the following may be seen.

- Cardiac enlargement.
- Upper lobe vascular prominence: from raised pulmonary venous pressure.

- Pleural effusions: seen as blunting at the costophrenic angles, but as the effusions become larger there is a homogeneous basal opacity with a concave upper border.
- Interstitial pulmonary oedema: initially, prominence of the upper lobe and narrowing of the lower lobe vessels. As venous pressure rises, interstitial oedema develops and fluid accumulates in the *interlobular areas* with peripheral septal lines (Kerley 'B' lines).
- Alveolar pulmonary oedema. With further increases in venous pressure, fluid transgresses into the alveolar spaces (alveolar shadowing) with haziness and blurring in the perihilar regions; in severe cases, pulmonary oedema develops throughout both lung fields. The outer thirds of the lungs may be spared, the bilateral central oedema being described as 'bat's wing'.

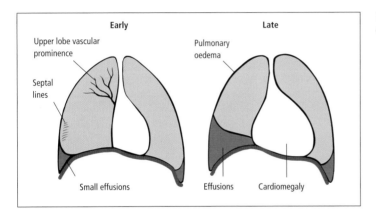

Figure 3.17 Manifestations of cardiac failure.

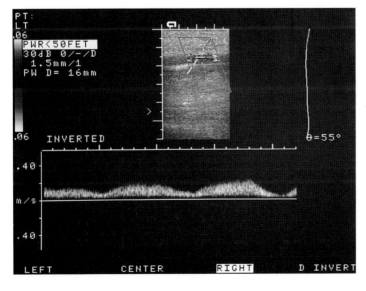

Figure 3.18 Doppler examination of the femoral vein with a normal Doppler signal and blood flow.

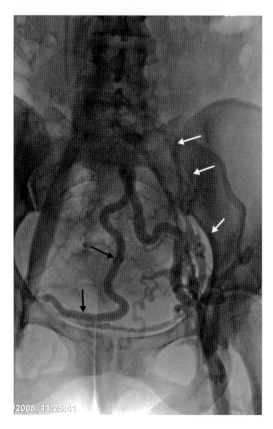

Figure 3.19 Left iliac vein thrombosis (white arrows) giving rise to collateral circulation to the right femoral vein (black arrows).

Deep vein thrombosis

Thrombus formation in the deep veins of the calf is a common clinical problem. Predisposing causes include recent surgery, contraceptive use, prolonged bed rest, neoplastic disease and hypercoagulability states.

Presentation

- Calf swelling.
- Calf pain.

- Pulmonary embolus may be the first sign, the calves being asymptomatic.

Radiological investigations

- Colour Doppler ultrasound.
- Venography.

Radiological features

Colour Doppler ultrasound is the initial investigation of choice but difficulty may be encountered in visualizing calf veins, especially in obese patients. If there is a strong clinical suspicion, in the presence of a normal Doppler examination, venography is suggested.

- *Colour Doppler ultrasound.* Accurately images vascular flow patterns and the presence of thrombus in the lower limbs. Blood clot may be seen within the vein lumen, often accompanied by a reduction in blood flow.
- *Venography.* Contrast injected into a foot vein visualizes the lower limb circulation, thrombus being seen as filling defects in the vein lumen. Extensive thrombus formation may lead to poor or complete lack of venous filling.

Complications

- Pulmonary embolus.
- Postphlebitic syndrome.

Treatment

- Heparin.
- Anticoagulants.
- Vena cava filter insertion in recurrent pulmonary embolization. Introduced percutaneously via the femoral or internal jugular vein and positioned in the IVC, just below the renal veins.

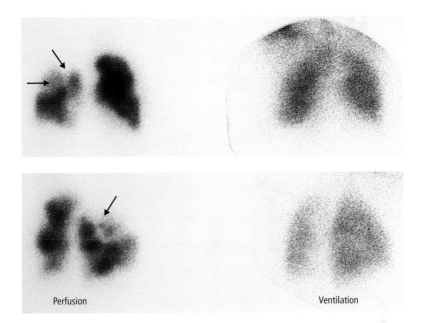

Perfusion   Ventilation

Figure 3.20 Perfusion and ventilation isotope scans in both the frontal and oblique projections showing mismatched defects suggesting pulmonary emboli.

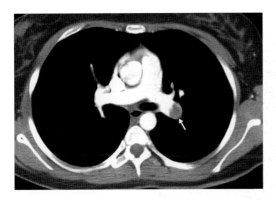

Figure 3.21 CT pulmonary angiogram showing embolus in the left main pulmonary artery (arrow).

Pulmonary embolus

Pulmonary embolism occurs when a blood clot detaches from the peripheral venous system and lodges in the pulmonary artery or its branches.

Pulmonary infarction is the lesion that develops secondary to pulmonary embolus.

Predisposing causes include prolonged bed rest, surgery, recent air travel, pregnancy, hypercoagulable states and lower limb deep vein thrombosis.

Radiological features

The blood clot usually originates from the pelvic or lower limb veins and migrates into the pulmonary circulation. The chest X-ray is often normal, but if pulmonary infarction develops, any of the following may be seen:

- raised diaphragm;
- small pleural effusions;
- basal collapse or plate-like atelectasis;
- consolidation, often segmental, peripherally situated and wedge-shaped.

Isotope scan

Pulmonary embolus results in a segmental defect in perfusion with preserved ventilation (ventilation/perfusion mismatch).

CT pulmonary arteriography (CTPA)

A rapid series of scans are taken through the lungs after intravenous injection of a large bolus of contrast; emboli are seen as filling defects in the contrast column.

Pulmonary angiography

Now uncommonly preformed; direct contrast injection into the pulmonary arteries reveals blood clot as intraluminal filling defects with obstruction and attenuation of the pulmonary arterial branches. Infusion of thrombolytics through the catheter may lyse the clot.

Complications

Pulmonary hypertension: resolves in the acute stage when thrombi disintegrate. However, it may persist with recurrent embolization.

Types of embolism

- *Fat embolism.* Usually seen after severe skeletal trauma with fat globules entering the circulation and obstructing pulmonary vessels.
- *Septic embolism.* Arising from tricuspid endocarditis or infected material from central venous pressure (CVP) lines, pacing wires, etc.
- *Amniotic fluid embolism.* Commonest cause of postpartum maternal death. Amniotic debris may gain access to the maternal circulation with subsequent embolization.

> **Key point**
>
> CT pulmonary angiography is an accurate method of detecting pulmonary emboli

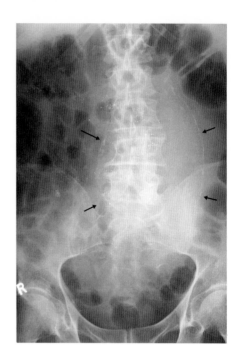

Figure 3.22 Plain abdominal film showing curvilinear calcification (arrows) in a large abdominal aortic aneurysm.

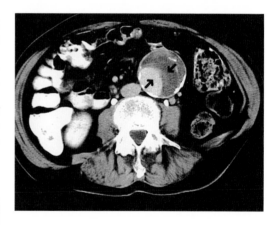

Figure 3.23 CT abdomen after contrast shows filling of the lumen (↗) and thrombus in an aneurysm (↙).

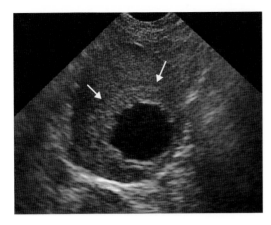

Figure 3.24 Transverse ultrasound of the abdomen showing the lumen (black) surrounded by thrombus (arrows).

Abdominal aortic aneurysm

An aneurysm refers to a localized dilatation of the vessel wall. Aneurysms may arise in any part of the aorta, but are most frequently seen in the abdominal aorta below the level of the renal arteries. Degenerative vascular disease with subsequent weakening of the vessel wall is the usual cause.

Presentation

Asymptomatic finding; abdominal pain or back pain from vertebral erosion; pulsatile abdominal mass; acute abdomen.

Radiological features

- *Plain abdominal films* may show curvilinear calcification in the wall of an aneurysm, especially when due to atherosclerosis. Calcification is more clearly visualized on a lateral abdominal film.
- *Ultrasound* is the best initial investigation to determine the presence of an aneurysm, measure its diameter and assess subsequent progress. An increased threat of rupture exists with those >6 cm in diameter and elective surgery is recommended.
- *CT* and *MRI* are both useful to localize the exact site of an aneurysm; assessment of renal artery involvement is essential to determine the type of operative approach.
- *Arteriography*: abdominal aneurysms may not necessarily show a widened lumen as the majority contain thrombus. Arteriography will demonstrate the distal circulation and relation of the renal arteries to the aneurysm.

Types of aneurysm

- Traumatic.
- Congenital: most commonly affects the intracranial circulation in the region of the circle of Willis ('berry aneurysm').
- Inflammatory: infection or abscess around the aorta leads to weakening of the wall.
- Dissecting: usually due to a tear in a weakened intimal wall in the thoracic aorta; predisposing factors include hypertension and Marfan syndrome. Retrograde dissection can involve the coronary arteries, aortic valve and the pericardial sac. CT or MRI may detect an intimal flap separating the two lumina, MRI being the more sensitive investigation.
- Degenerative: commonest sites are the abdominal aorta, iliacs, femorals and popliteals.
- Poststenotic: distal to arterial narrowing, such as coarctation.

> **Key point**
>
> Abdominal aneurysm measuring more than 5.5 cm in diameter needs treatment, either surgical or endovascular stenting

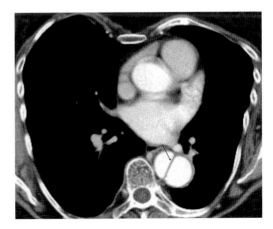

Figure 3.25 Aortic dissection.

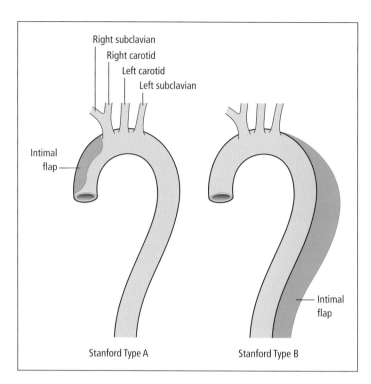

Figure 3.26 Types of dissection.

Right subclavian
Right carotid
Left carotid
Left subclavian

Intimal flap

Intimal flap

Stanford Type A

Stanford Type B

Aortic dissection

Aortic dissection results in a tear in the aortic wall where blood penetrates the intima and enters the media layer, forcing the layers apart.

Presentation

- Sudden onset of severe pain – anterior or posterior chest, often interscapular.
- Neurological deficit if aortic root vessels involved, myocardial infarction, upper limb paraplegia, limb ischaemia, and bowel ischaemia.

Predisposing causes

- Hypertension.
- Pregnancy.
- Chest trauma.

- Connective tissue disorders.
- Increased incidence with bicuspid aortic valve.

Radiology

- Chest X-ray may show widened mediastinum or pleural effusion.
- MRI, with no radiation or contrast administration needed.
- CT – shows intimal flap separating true and false lumen.
- Transoesophageal echocardiography, which can be carried out at bedside.
- Aortography, now rarely used.

Treatment

- Control blood pressure.
- Ascending aortic dissection usually requires surgical management.
- Descending aorta dissection can be medically managed, unless there is vascular compromise of vital visceral structures.

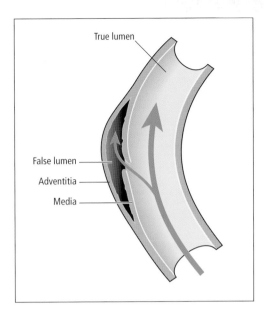

Figure 3.27 Mechanism of dissection.

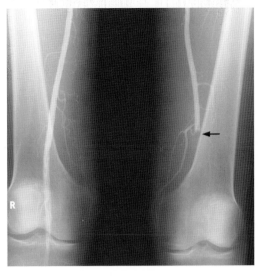

Figure 3.29 Femoral embolus: sharp contrast cut-off in the left femoral artery (arrow) due to embolus. Note the poor collateral circulation.

Peripheral vascular disease

Arterial insufficiency commonly develops in the lower limbs from atheromatous involvement of the aorta and lower limb arteries. Pain in the calves or buttocks on exercise (intermittent claudication), cold limbs and ulceration are the commonest clinical features. Predisposing causes include diabetes and smoking.

Radiological investigations

Doppler ultrasound; arteriography; MRI.

Radiological features

- Ultrasound will diagnose major occlusions, but arteriography is required for the accurate visualization of diseased vessels, stenoses and occlusions.
- MR angiography has shown significant improvements and is a valuable additional modality for diagnosis.

Treatment

- Balloon angioplasty.
- Metallic stent insertion under radiological control.
- Surgical bypass grafts: aorto-iliac, femoropopliteal and femorofemoral.

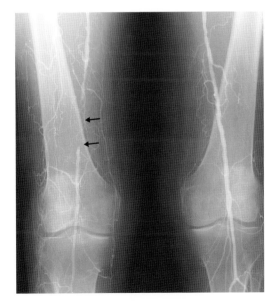

Figure 3.28 Arteriogram: occluded segment (arrows) in the right femoral artery.

Arterial embolus

An arterial embolus occurs when a blood clot, originating elsewhere in the cardiovascular system, travels more peripherally and occludes an artery. The lower limbs are affected in the majority of cases. Symptoms are of rapid onset and consist of a cold, pale, numb leg with absent pulses distal to the occlusion. Predisposing factors include recent myocardial infarction with mural thrombus and atrial fibrillation. If there is coexisting vascular disease, a diagnosis of acute thrombosis should be considered.

Radiological features

Peripheral arteriography demonstrates the contrast column in the artery with a sharp, well-defined cut-off point, usually a convex upper border projecting into the lumen of the vessel. Further evidence of an acute episode is provided by a deficient collateral circulation.

Treatment

- Surgical embolectomy.
- Thrombolysis: perfusion of streptokinase or tissue plasminogen activator (TPA) directly into the arterial thrombus in order to lyse the clot.

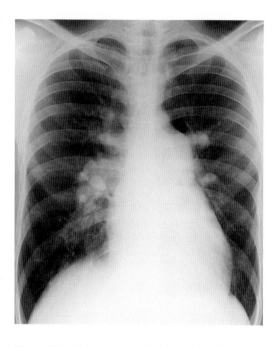

Figure 3.30 Pulmonary hypertension: bilateral hilar vascular enlargement and prominence of the pulmonary outflow tract.

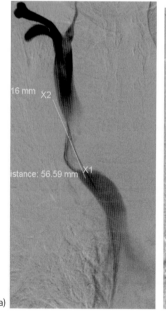 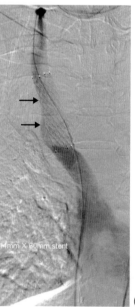

(a) (b)

Figure 3.31 (a) Significant narrowing of the SVC leading to obstruction; (b) SVC stent in place (arrows).

Pulmonary arterial hypertension

Pulmonary arterial hypertension refers to increased pulmonary artery pressure from its normal value of 25/10 mmHg to greater than 30/15 mmHg.

Radiological features

Hypertension has to be quite marked before changes are seen on a chest X-ray.

- Cardiac enlargement with right ventricular hypertrophy.
- Dilatation of the pulmonary hilar vessels with distal attenuation.
- Distension of the main pulmonary artery with a bulge below the aortic knuckle.

Causes

- Increased pulmonary blood flow in congenital heart disease.
- Obstruction of the pulmonary circulation, e.g. pulmonary emboli, parenchymal lung disease.
- Secondary to pulmonary venous hypertension from left-heart failure or mitral stenosis.

Superior and inferior vena cava obstruction

The SVC and IVC may obstruct from many causes resulting in distal venous distension.

Presentation

- SVC obstruction: facial and neck oedema, visible collateral veins.
- IVC obstruction: lower limb oedema, scrotal oedema.

Radiological investigations

- *Doppler ultrasound*: verifies decreased or lack of a blood flow pattern.
- *CT/MRI*: confirms occlusion and often identifies the cause.

- *Venography*: demonstrates anatomical detail, especially useful if stenting is to be considered.

Causes of SVC obstruction

- Neoplastic: bronchial carcinoma, lymphoma, radiotherapy.
- Benign: mediastinal disease due to tuberculosis, sarcoid.

Causes of IVC obstruction

- Tumour invasion from abdominal neoplasms, most commonly renal.
- Retroperitoneal fibrosis; radiotherapy.

> **Key point**
>
> In acute SVC obstruction from malignant thoracic disease, consider SVC stenting

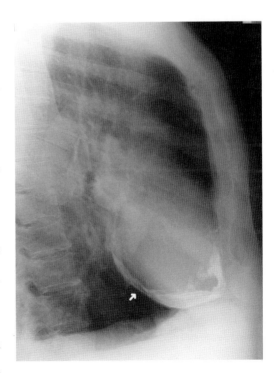

Figure 3.32 Pericardial calcification (arrow).

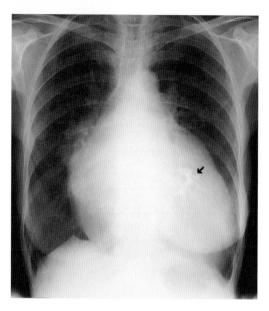

Figure 3.33 Enlarged heart resulting from mitral valvular disease showing valve calcification (arrow).

Cardiac calcification

Pericardial calcification

May follow pericarditis, tuberculosis, rheumatoid arthritis, rheumatic fever and pyogenic or viral pericarditis; the aetiology may be unknown.

Myocardial calcification

Occurs typically at the apex of the left ventricle; common causes are myocardial infarction and ventricular aneurysm.

Valve calcification

Calcification in the valves is common, but has to be quite extensive before being evident on plain films. Calcification usually means an element of stenosis, with the aortic and mitral valves most commonly affected. Causes include atheroma, rheumatic valvular disease and congenital bicuspid valve.

Aortic wall calcification

May be present in atheroma, in the wall of an aneurysm or represent syphilitic aortitis (ascending aorta).

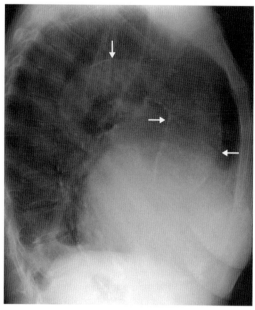

Figure 3.34 Aortic-wall calcification (arrows).

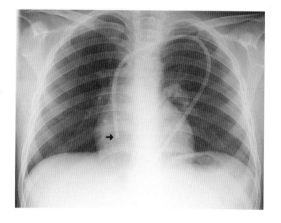

Figure 3.35 Tip of the central line in the right atrium (arrow).

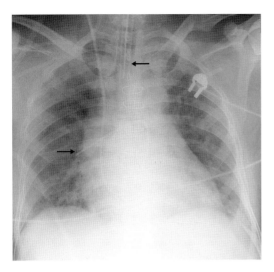

Figure 3.36 Swan-Ganz catheter in the right pulmonary artery (→) and endotracheal tube (←) in a patient after cardiac surgery (note ECG leads).

Tube and catheter placement

Endotracheal tube

The tip should be positioned 5–7 cm above the carina. When sited too distally into the trachea, the endotracheal tube may advance into a main bronchus, causing collapse of the opposite lung.

Central line

Inserted via the jugular or subclavian veins into a large intrathoracic vein. For accurate measurement of right atrial pressure, the tip of the catheter must lie in a large intrathoracic vein such as the SVC.

Swan-Ganz catheter

The catheter is inserted via the jugular, subclavian or femoral vein and manipulated through the right heart into either the right or left pulmonary artery. The end-diastolic left-ventricular pressure is estimated from a reading taken at the distal tip of the catheter.

Nasogastric tube

The radiopaque tip should be visualized in the region of the stomach on plain films. An X-ray is usually necessary to ensure that the tube is not malpositioned, especially into the trachea or bronchus.

Pacing wire

Pacemaker leads are placed through the subclavian or internal jugular veins into the right side of the heart, with the tip implanted at the apex of the right ventricle, whereas dual lead pacemakers have their ends positioned in the right atrium and ventricle.

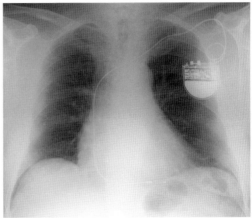

Figure 3.37 Single pacing lead.

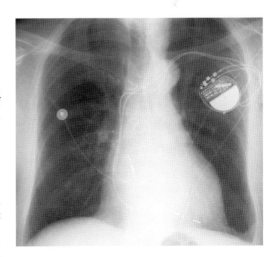

Figure 3.38 Dual pacing leads.

4

Gastrointestinal tract

Gastrointestinal tract investigations

Plain films

Plain films may be helpful in detecting intestinal obstruction, extraluminal free gas and abdominal calcification.

Sialography

This examination may be indicated in the investigation of a parotid or submandibular calculus or swelling. Contrast is injected into the orifice of the parotid or submandibular duct; calculi in the main ducts appear as filling defects in the contrast column.

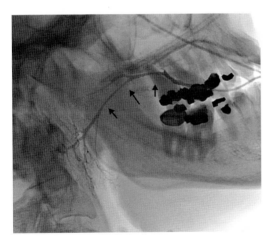

Figure 4.1 Parotid sialogram with contrast injection into the parotid duct (arrows).

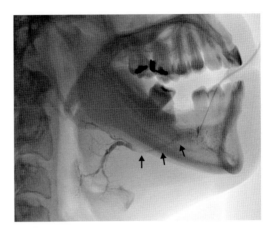

Figure 4.2 Submandibular sialogram. Contrast injection into the submandibular duct (arrows).

Barium swallow

Barium sulphate is used for most contrast examinations of the gastrointestinal tract. Water-soluble agents are preferred in situations where a perforation is suspected as extraluminal barium is potentially hazardous. The main indications are dysphagia and symptoms of gastro-oesophageal reflux. The oesophagus is visualized under fluoroscopy as the patient swallows barium and studied for incoordinate peristalsis, motility problems or structural abnormalities. For pharyngeal disorders, real-time imaging is helpful.

Barium meal

Endoscopy is the preferred examination to visualize the stomach, but barium studies may occasionally be useful for the elderly or those who cannot tolerate endoscopy.

Radiology: Lecture Notes, Fourth Edition. Pradip R. Patel.
© 2020 John Wiley & Sons Ltd. Published 2020 by John Wiley & Sons Ltd.
Companion website: www.wiley.com/go/patel/radiology

After an overnight fast, barium and effervescent powders are given under fluoroscopy. Images are obtained in different projections. The gastro-oesophageal junction is observed for reflux.

Barium follow-through

Transit of barium is observed through the small bowel after 200–300 ml of barium is swallowed. Full-length abdominal images are taken every half hour until the barium reaches the terminal ileum and large bowel. Specific images of the terminal ileum are obtained.

Gastrograffin

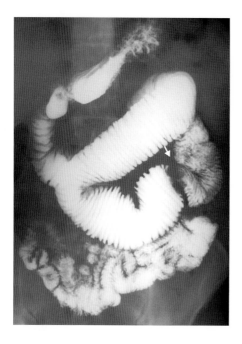

Figure 4.3 Barium follow-through: small bowel stricture with significant proximal bowel dilation in a partial small bowel obstruction (arrow).

Small bowel enema

A tube is passed nasally and manoeuvred into the duodenojejunal flexure under fluoroscopic control. Subsequently, dilute barium is infused until a continuous column of barium reaches the terminal ileum. The technique is more rapid and exact in the detection of small bowel pathology than a barium follow-through examination, although more unpleasant for the patient.

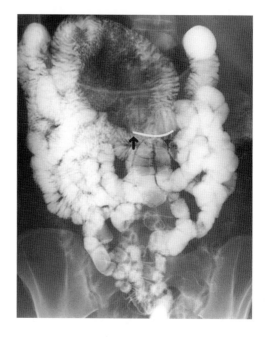

Figure 4.4 Normal small bowel enema. Note the tip of the tube in the jejunum (arrow).

Barium enema

Colonoscopy is now the investigation of choice to examine the large bowel, having the advantage of being able to remove most polyps and also to carry out biopsy procedures.

Barium enema examinations have declined significantly in importance and are now rarely carried out.

A clean colon is essential and laxatives are administered the day before the examination. Barium is run into the colon by means of a tube placed in the rectum and images are obtained under fluoroscopic control. Air introduced into the large bowel produces a double-contrast examination. A rare, recognized complication is bowel perforation, which may result in peritonitis.

Isotope scanning

Technetium-99m pertechnetate may be used for studies of gastric emptying and also in the detection of a Meckel's diverticulum (accumulation in ectopic gastric mucosa). It may diagnose the source of a gastrointestinal haemorrhage; it is not site specific but it can detect haemorrhage at lower levels of bleeding (0.1 ml/second) than other techniques can.

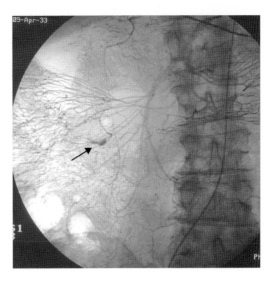

Figure 4.6 Superior mesenteric angiogram; extravasated contrast in severe colonic haemorrhage (arrow).

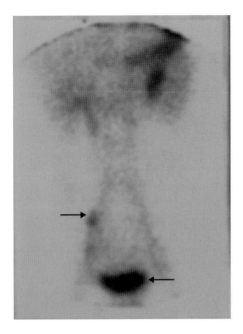

Figure 4.5 Isotope scan showing accumulation in a Meckel's diverticulum (→). The larger area at the bottom is the bladder (←).

Arteriography

Selective visceral angiography with contrast injection into the superior and inferior mesenteric arteries may pinpoint the source of acute small or large bowel haemorrhage. Additionally, the bleeding may be stopped by the infusion of vasoconstrictors or embolic materials; however, in order to detect bleeding, it has to be fairly brisk at approximately 0.5–1.0 ml/min. Other indications for angiography include identifying islet cell tumours of the pancreas, evaluating bowel ischaemia and pancreatic tumour resectability.

Computed tomography (CT) scanning

Uses in the gastrointestinal tract include:

- to assess for operability by staging oesophageal, gastric and colonic tumours for adjacent infiltration and secondary deposits;
- localizing abscesses and postoperative complications;
- as an aid to biopsy and drainage procedures.

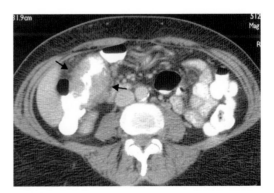

Figure 4.7 CT abdomen showing an ascending colon carcinoma (arrows).

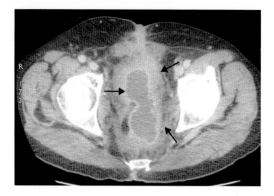

Figure 4.8 CT pelvis: large pelvic abscess following colonic surgery (arrows).

- CT colonography for large bowel lesions. Air is introduced into the colon via a rectal catheter and CT images are taken of the abdomen. Meticulous preparation of the colon is necessary as faecal residue can be misinterpreted as a polyp.

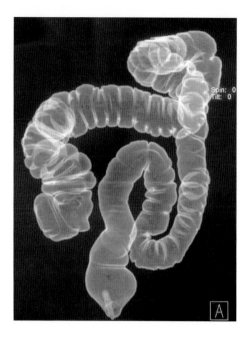

Figure 4.10 CT pneumocolon. CT of the abdomen with special reconstructions of the colon.

- MRI is now increasingly more useful in small bowel studies, especially as there is no radiation involved.

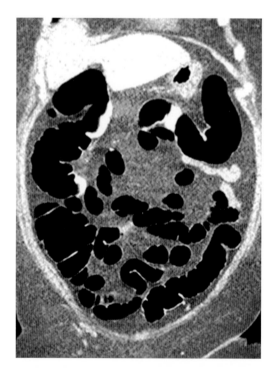

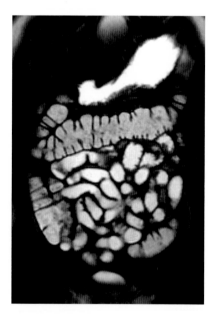

Figure 4.9 CT colonography with air insufflation in a well-prepared colon.

Figure 4.11 MRI normal small bowel study demonstrating the jejunum and ileum.

Plain abdomen film

The routine projection used is the supine one. Erect abdomen films may illustrate air/fluid levels in obstruction and free gas under the diaphragm in perforation, although an erect chest film is more useful to visualize free gas.

When assessing an abdominal film, a study of three principal aspects will encompass the majority of abnormal findings: bowel gas pattern; areas of calcification; skeletal abnormalities.

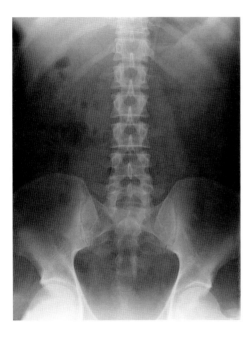

Figure 4.12 Normal plain abdomen.

Bowel gas pattern

- Marked variation exists in the amount of bowel gas in normal individuals, usually some gas being noted in the stomach, small and large bowel.
- Bowel gas pattern should be evaluated with particular reference to dilatation. Small bowel dilatation is considered to be present if the width exceeds 3 cm.
- Generally, the small bowel lies in a central position characterized by folds or valvulae conniventes forming complete bands across the bowel.
- The large bowel is situated peripherally, the haustral pattern forming incomplete transverse bands.
- Conditions that may be diagnosed by alteration in the bowel gas pattern are small bowel obstruction, large bowel obstruction, paralytic ileus, caecal volvulus, sigmoid volvulus and toxic megacolon.
- Gas may be noted outside the bowel lumen in the biliary system, urinary tract, subphrenic abscess, colon wall or abdominal abscess.

Calcification

A great majority of calcifications are of no real clinical significance: costal cartilage, pelvic vein phleboliths, mesenteric lymph nodes and vascular calcification. Some abnormal areas are shown in the figure below.

Skeletal abnormalities

Skeletal abnormalities that may be shown on plain abdominal films are: degenerative changes in the spine or hips; bony metastases; Paget's disease; sacroiliitis; vertebral body collapse.

Other abnormalities

Hepatosplenomegaly; mass lesions seen by distortion of the bowel gas pattern; soft-tissue masses arising from intra-abdominal and pelvic organs.

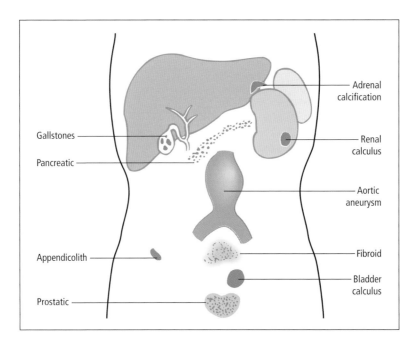

Figure 4.13 Pathological calcifications in the abdomen.

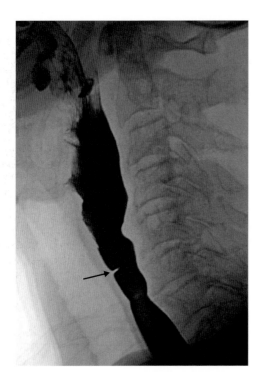

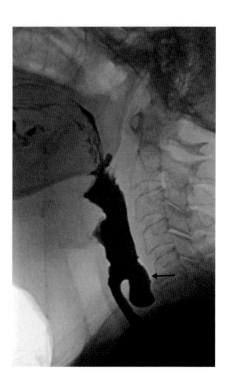

Figure 4.14 Barium swallow: oesophageal web (arrow).   Figure 4.15 Barium swallow: pharyngeal pouch (arrow).

Oesophageal web

An oesophageal web is a thin membranous band arising from the anterior upper oesophageal wall, especially from the pharyngo-oesophageal junction. It is covered with normal-appearing mucosa and protrudes posteriorly to a varying extent. Webs may be multiple and there is a recognized association with postcricoid carcinoma.

Presentation

Dysphagia; incidental finding; iron-deficiency anaemia (Plummer–Vinson syndrome).

Radiological features

Barium study reveals an anterior fine linear filling defect on the barium-filled upper oesophagus. Webs are best seen on the lateral projection.

Treatment

Oesophagoscopy usually ruptures the web and also excludes other oesophageal pathology.

> **Key point**
>
> Webs may be incidental and not always associated with symptoms

Pharyngeal pouch

A pharyngeal pouch results from a posterior mucosal protrusion arising from between the vertical and horizontal fibres of the inferior constrictor of the pharynx, just above the cricopharyngeus. Lateral pouches or diverticula are rare. Diverticula may be found in any part of the oesophagus; aspiration pneumonia is a recognized complication.

Presentation

Dysphagia; repeated attacks of aspiration pneumonia; food regurgitation; halitosis; palpable neck mass.

Radiological features

Plain films of the cervical region in the erect position may show a fluid level in the pouch. A barium swallow reveals the pouch filling posteriorly from the oesophageal wall, connected by a relatively narrow neck and often containing stagnating food residue.

Treatment

Surgical resection, using an external approach or by endoscopic technique.

> **Key point**
>
> Aspiration pneumonia is an important complication of a pouch

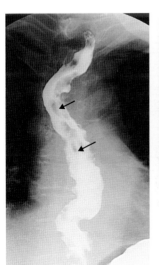 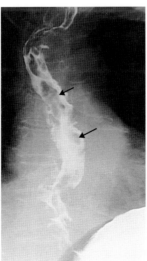

Figure 4.16 Varices: serpiginous filling defects in the oesophagus (arrows).

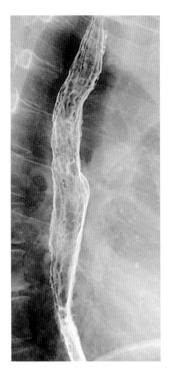 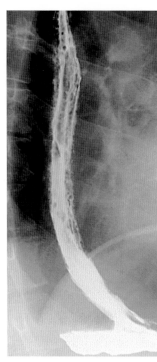

Figure 4.17 Irregular mucosal outline in monilial infection.

Oesophageal varices

Oesophageal varices are venous anastomotic collateral veins, usually resulting from portal venous hypertension or portal vein obstruction. They commonly develop as a result of liver cirrhosis, are confined to the lower two-thirds of the oesophagus and are often associated with gastric varices ('uphill varices' with portosystemic shunting: collateral blood flow via the azygos vein into the superior vena cava (SVC) from the portal vein). Varices in the upper oesophagus can develop from SVC obstruction ('downhill varices': collaterals from SVC, via azygos vein into inferior vena cava (IVC) or the portal vein).

Radiological features

- Endoscopy is the investigation of choice but a barium swallow may delineate the large submucosal veins in the oesophagus and gastric fundus in many cases.
- On the barium-filled column, varices are seen as serpiginous tortuous filling defects.

- Contrast-enhanced CT scanning may also identify varices and the portal vein.

Moniliasis

Fungal infection of the oesophagus with *Candida* occurs in patients who are debilitated, immunosuppressed or on broad-spectrum antibiotic therapy. The incidence of pharyngeal and oesophageal candidiasis is particularly high in patients with acquired immune deficiency syndrome (AIDS).

Presentation

Painful dysphagia; chest pain.

Radiological features

- On barium swallow examination, the margins of the oesophagus are irregular with small mucosal plaques, seen as filling defects.
- The mucosa may be ulcerated with a cobblestone appearance.

Differential of an irregular oesophagus

- Oesophagitis following caustic ingestion: in the acute stage, atonic, ulcerated oesophagus with subsequent stricture formation.
- Reflux oesophagitis.
- Herpetic oesophagitis.

> **Key point**
>
> Oesophageal moniliasis almost always occurs in immunocompromised patients

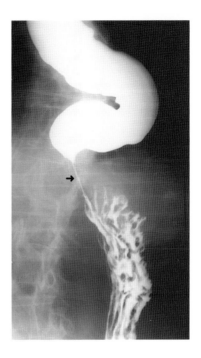

Figure 4.19 Achalasia: dilated tortuous oesophagus with narrowing at the gastro-oesophageal junction (arrow).

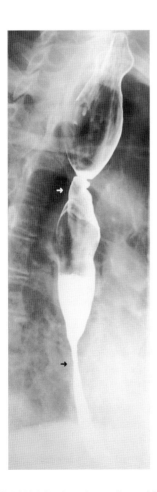

Figure 4.18 Multiple benign strictures (arrows) from caustic soda ingestion; the mucosal outline appears smooth.

Benign oesophageal stricture

Benign oesophageal strictures have numerous aetiologies, and often present with dysphagia. Carcinoma should always be suspected in the presence of an oesophageal stricture, as radiological appearances can sometimes be misleading.

Radiological features

- Acute stage – there may be oedema and ulceration of the oesophagus.
- Chronic benign strictures have smooth tapering margins, often with proximal dilatation.

Causes

The usual cause is peptic stricture secondary to reflux; others include:

- corrosive stricture: tend to be long and smooth in the chronic phase;
- achalasia: found at the level of the diaphragm;
- skin disorders: epidermolysis bullosa and pemphigus;
- traumatic: from prolonged indwelling nasogastric tube;
- radiotherapy;
- scleroderma.

Achalasia

Achalasia is a functional disorder of motility secondary to an abnormality of the Auerbach plexus, which causes an inability of the lower oesophageal sphincter to relax. Dysphagia, weight loss and regurgitation of stagnating oesophageal contents are the commonest presenting symptoms. Complications include recurrent pulmonary aspiration and an increased incidence of oesophageal carcinoma.

Radiological features

- *Chest film*: the dilated oesophagus may be rendered visible by retained food contents giving rise to a widened mediastinum. Reduced air in the stomach produces a small or absent gastric air bubble. Aspiration into the lungs may lead to chronic basal changes.
- *Barium swallow*: shows gross oesophageal dilatation and tortuosity, usually with retained food residue. There is poor peristaltic activity, with narrowing at the oesophagogastric junction due to failure of relaxation of the lower sphincter.

Treatment

- Local injection of Botulinum toxin at the narrowed segment.
- Balloon dilatation in the narrowed segment to rupture the muscle fibres.
- Oesophagomyotomy (Heller's operation).

Key point

There is an increased incidence of oesophageal carcinoma in achalasia

---

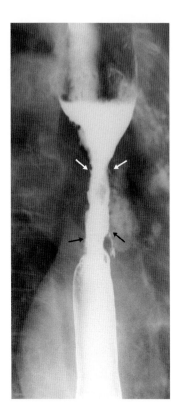

Figure 4.20 Contrast swallow showing an oesophageal carcinoma with irregular narrowing and mucosal destruction (arrows).

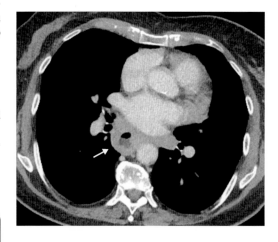

Figure 4.21 CT thorax: oesophageal thickening due to a carcinoma (arrow).

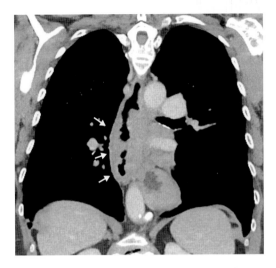

Figure 4.22 Coronal CT showing a large oesophageal carcinoma (arrows).

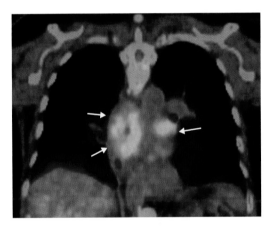

Figure 4.23 PET scan showing uptake in the oesophageal carcinoma (arrows) with spread to the left hilum (arrow).

Oesophageal carcinoma

Carcinoma of the oesophagus, usually a squamous cell type, occurs most frequently in the distal third of the oesophagus and is more common in males. Predisposing factors include achalasia, Barrett's oesophagus (columnar epithelium lining the oesophagus), caustic stricture and the Plummer–Vinson syndrome.

Presentation

- Progressive dysphagia, often painful.
- Weight loss.

Radiological investigations

- *Barium swallow*: the initial investigation of choice.
- *CT scanning thorax*: assesses tumour confinement to the wall or extraluminal spread into the adjacent mediastinum and secondary spread to supraclavicular nodes.
- *CT scanning abdomen or ultrasound abdomen*: to search for secondary deposits in the liver and para-aortic nodes.

Radiological features

On barium examination.

- Polypoidal type: intraluminal mass protrudes into the oesophageal lumen causing a filling defect in the barium column.
- Infiltrative type: tumour spread under the oesophageal mucosa causes narrowing. Subsequent mucosal infiltration results in ulceration and irregular oesophageal outline. Occasionally, there is a tracheo- or broncho-oesophageal fistula.

Treatment

For patients with early tumours limited to the mucosa, five-year survival can be higher than 80%, but presentation is often late leading to poor outcome as most have mediastinal or distant spread; therapy is then often palliative.

- Surgical resection: when there is no mediastinal or distant spread. A postoperative check of the integrity of the anastomosis can be made with a water-soluble contrast swallow examination.
- Palliative radiotherapy: squamous cell carcinomas are responsive with rapid relief of symptoms.
- Palliative intubation: metallic stent insertion under fluoroscopic control.

> **Key point**
>
> Reflux in Barrett's oesophagus is a predisposing cause of oesophageal carcinoma

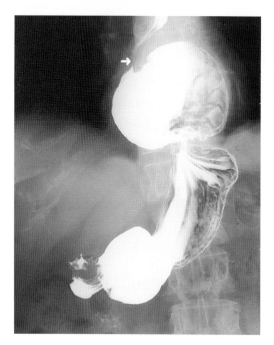

Figure 4.24 Sliding hiatus hernia: the gastro-oesopha-geal junction (arrow) is above the diaphragm.

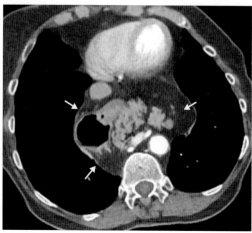

Figure 4.26 CT scan showing a large hiatus hernia posterior to the heart containing stomach and bowel (arrows).

Hiatus hernia

A hiatus hernia develops from protrusion of a portion of the stomach, through the oesophageal hiatus of the diaphragm, into the thorax. A broad spectrum of appearances arises, ranging from the whole stomach lying in the intrathoracic position to small hernia-tions, which slide back easily.

Sliding hiatus hernia

The most common type, where the gastro-oesophageal junction and the stomach slide to lie above the diaphragm, often with associated gastro-oesophageal reflux. The hernia is usually reducible in the erect position.

Para-oesophageal hernia

The gastro-oesophageal junction lies in a normal position with the stomach herniating alongside the oesophagus. It is uncommon and usually irreducible, without associated reflux.

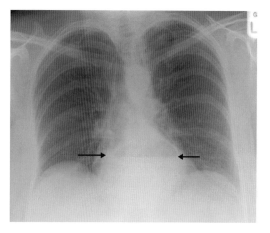

Figure 4.25 Chest X-ray showing a large hiatus hernia with a fluid level overlying the cardiac shadow (arrows).

Presentation

- Heartburn: worse on lying flat.
- Dysphagia: due to either inflammatory change or stricture.
- Retrosternal pain: can be mistaken for cardiac pain.
- Anaemia.

Radiological features

- *Chest X-ray*: may demonstrate a soft-tissue mass in the posterior mediastinum, behind the cardiac shadow. An air/fluid level is sometimes noted in the hernia.
  - CT – A hiatus hernia is readily seen on CT examination, often as an incidental finding during investigations for chest or abdominal pathologies.
- *Barium swallow*: readily shows the herniation. The patient needs to be examined in the 'head-down' position to demonstrate small herniations with or without gastro-oesophageal reflux.

Complications

- Oesophagitis: inflammatory changes secondary to acid regurgitation.
- Oesophageal ulceration: associated with reflux.
- Oesophageal stricture: healing by fibrosis can lead to stricture formation. When this complication arises, an endoscopy is needed to exclude a stricture secondary to carcinoma.
- Anaemia.
- Incarceration, though rare, may lead to obstruction, perforation, strangulation, haemorrhage or respiratory symptoms.

Gastric outlet obstruction

Gastric outlet obstruction occurs when there is a mechanical obstruction at the outlet of the stomach at the level of the pylorus or duodenum. The stomach often dilates to accommodate food intake and secretions.

Presentation

Vomiting, weight loss and electrolyte imbalance from persistent vomiting.

Investigations

- Endoscopy.
- CT.
- Barium studies.

Radiological features

- CT demonstrates the distended stomach and often a cause such as a gastric or pancreatic tumour.
- Contrast studies are now not often used but may show a distended often enlarged stomach, the presence of food residue, delay in emptying, diminished peristaltic activity, and narrowing and irregularity of the gastric outlet, from fibrosis or malignant infiltration.

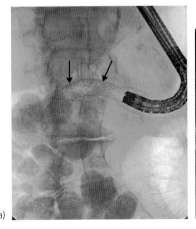 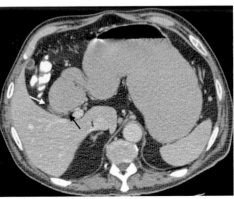

(a) (b)

Figure 4.27 (a) Pyloric stent in place (arrows) to relieve malignant obstruction; (b) CT abdomen: grossly dilated stomach in gastric outlet obstruction (arrows).

Treatment

- Operative; resection of obstructing lesion.
- Palliative; endoscopic self-expandable metal stenting.

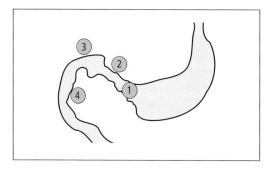

Figure 4.28 Causes of gastric outlet obstruction. 1, Gastric antrum: ulcer or carcinoma; 2, pyloric canal: adult hypertrophic stenosis (rare); 3, duodenal cap: ulceration with scarring of the duodenal cap; 4, duodenal loop: pancreatic carcinoma or duodenal carcinoma.

Key point

Pancreatic carcinoma is the commonest malignant cause of gastric outlet obstruction

---

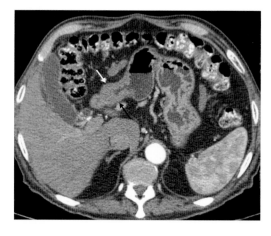

Figure 4.29 CT abdomen: carcinoma of the stomach – pyloric antrum (arrows).

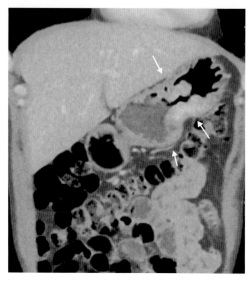

Figure 4.30 Gastric carcinoma with gastric wall thickening (arrows).

Gastric carcinoma

There has been a general decrease in the incidence of gastric carcinoma, although there remains a very high prevalence of the disease in the Japanese population. Predisposing factors include pernicious anaemia, chronic atrophic gastritis, adenomatous polyps, previous partial gastrectomy and *Helicobacter pylori* infection.

Presentation

Dyspepsia; anorexia; nausea and vomiting; weight loss; haematemesis or melaena.

Radiological investigations

- Endoscopy or barium meal.
- Ultrasound and CT for preoperative evaluation.

Radiological features

Barium meal examination may reveal the following forms of gastric carcinoma.

- Polypoidal type: soft-tissue mass causing a filling defect in the stomach.

- Ulcerating type: the ulcerating area is confined to within the margin of the stomach.
- Diffuse infiltrating type: diffuse submucosal infiltration with muscle invasion leads to a small, rigid stomach with poor distensibility: linitis plastica or 'leather bottle stomach'.
- Local infiltrating type: a focal area of mucosal irregularity and narrowing at the site of the tumour.

Treatment

At the time of diagnosis, gastric carcinoma is usually advanced, hence an extremely poor five-year survival rate. Treatment includes: total gastrectomy as a possible curative procedure; palliative chemotherapy and partial gastrectomy for obstruction.

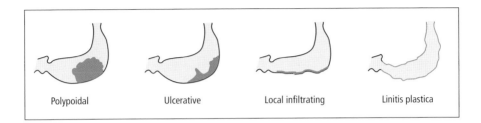

Polypoidal   Ulcerative   Local infiltrating   Linitis plastica

Figure 4.31 Types of gastric carcinoma.

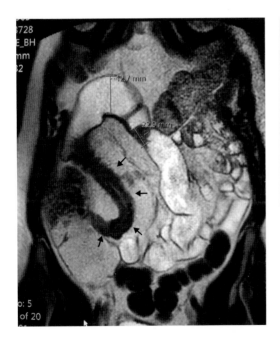

Figure 4.32 Small bowel MRI showing a long loop of ileum affected by Crohn's disease (arrows), causing obstruction with dilated proximal loop.

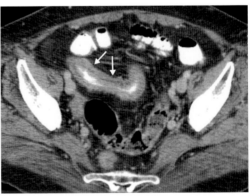

Figure 4.33 CT pelvis: marked thickening of the ileum in Crohn's disease (arrows).

Crohn's disease

Crohn's disease, a chronic inflammatory condition of unknown aetiology, can affect any part of the alimentary tract from the oesophagus to rectum, but most commonly involves the terminal ileum and small bowel.

Radiological features

The terminal ileum in the small bowel is the site most commonly affected, although the large bowel is also frequently affected and may be solely involved. On a barium follow-through study, the following small bowel abnormalities may be seen.

- Deep ulceration (rose thorn) affecting the entire bowel wall.
- Cobblestone mucosal appearance caused by ulcers separated by raised areas of oedema.
- Loss of peristalsis, thickening and rigidity of bowel wall; separation of small bowel loops due to the thickness of their walls.
- Stricture formation from oedema and fibrosis (string sign of Kantor). In colonic Crohn's disease, the most frequent features found are deep ulceration, aphthous ulcers and discontinuous involvement with normal intervening bowel (skip lesions). Capsule endoscopy is occasionally used.

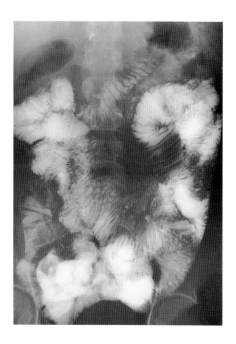

Figure 4.34 Malabsorption: contrast examination showing dilatation of small bowel with thickening of mucosal folds.

Complications

- Subacute obstruction as a result of stricture formation.
- Abscess formation, sometimes leading to bowel perforation.
- Malabsorption from extensive small bowel involvement and interruption of the enterohepatic circulation.
- Perianal inflammatory changes may result from abscess or fissure.
- Fistulae to large bowel, vagina, bladder, perineum and abdominal wall from inflamed small bowel adhering to adjacent structures.

Extrahepatic

Gallstones; sclerosing cholangitis; arthritis; oxalate and uric acid urinary calculi; uveitis.

Differential of small bowel narrowing

Adhesions; Crohn's disease; carcinoma (the duodenum is the most frequent site in the small bowel); metastases; radiotherapy; ischaemia; tuberculosis.

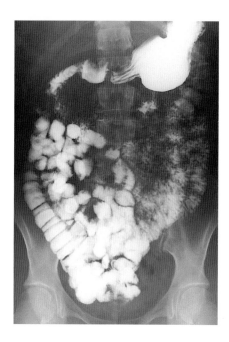

Figure 4.35 Normal barium follow-through examination of the small bowel. Barium has passed into the ascending colon.

Malabsorption

Malabsorption is characterized by a deficient intestinal absorption of essential nutrients.

Radiological features

Radiological examination of the small bowel is by barium follow-through examination. MRI scanning of the small bowel is proving to be a useful investigation.

Although causes such as Crohn's disease, fistulae or diverticula may be uncovered, the prime importance of radiology is to identify a malabsorption pattern. This is usually not specific for a diagnosis, and a jejunal biopsy may be required.

The following features may be shown on a barium examination:

- dilatation of small bowel;
- prominence of small bowel transverse bands, the valvulae conniventes;
- thickening of bowel wall, with separation of adjacent loops.

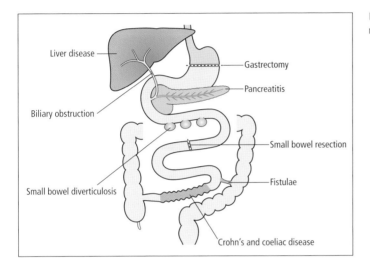

Figure 4.36 Causes of malabsorption.

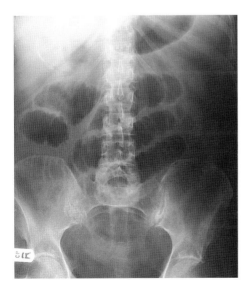

Figure 4.37 Small bowel obstruction: distended small bowel and absence of gas shadows in the colon.

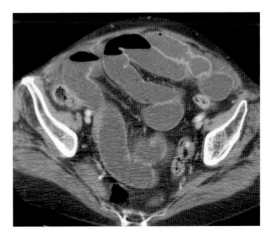

Figure 4.38 CT abdomen: dilated small bowel loops in small bowel obstruction.

Small bowel obstruction

Mechanical small bowel obstruction develops when there is impairment to the onward flow of bowel contents.

Radiological features

Gas and fluid accumulating proximal to the site of obstruction causes progressive dilatation of small bowel. Features on plain abdominal films include the following.

- Central distended loops of small bowel, often >3 cm in diameter.
- Transverse stripes of the valvulae conniventes generally extend across the whole of the small bowel; in the large bowel, the haustrae do not cross the colon.
- Absence of gas in the large bowel. If gas is still present, it indicates that obstruction is recent or that it is incomplete.
- When obstruction is high, such as the duodenum or upper jejunum, the above signs may be absent with lack of small bowel distension or fluid levels.
- The site of obstruction can be predicted. If only a few dilated loops are found, then the obstruction is likely to be upper jejunum, but a large number of small bowel loops indicates that obstruction is in the ileum: the greater the number of distended loops, the more distal the site of obstruction.

When plain abdominal films are equivocal, barium follow-through examination may identify the level of obstruction, the principal feature being a change in the calibre from the dilated segment to a collapsed distal small bowel. Barium should only be used if a colonic cause of obstruction has been excluded, as inspissated barium can turn an incomplete into a complete large bowel obstruction.

> **Key point**
>
> The level of small bowel obstruction can be judged by the number of distended small bowel loops

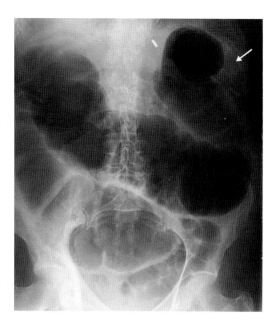

Figure 4.40 Large bowel obstruction with a distended colon up to the splenic flexure (arrow).

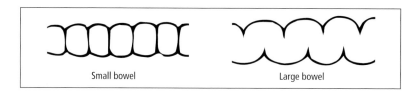

Small bowel   Large bowel

Figure 4.39 Appearance of valvulae conniventes in the small bowel and haustral pattern in the large bowel.

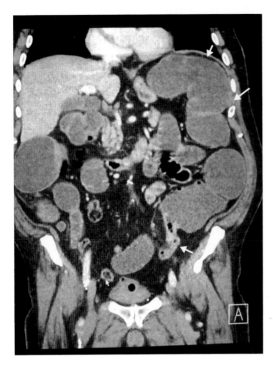

Figure 4.41 Coronal CT reconstruction showing sigmoid carcinoma (arrow) causing large bowel obstruction (arrows).

Large bowel obstruction

Obstruction of the large bowel usually results from either a colonic carcinoma (often rectosigmoid) or diverticular disease.

Radiological features

- Plain abdominal films show bowel distension.
- CT is accurate in identifying site and cause.
- Barium or water-soluble contrast enema is useful to confirm obstruction.

The basic principle is to detect bowel dilatation to a level beyond which there is collapse of bowel.

Features depend on the state of the ileocaecal valve.

- *With closed ileocaecal valve.* Gas distension is limited to large bowel. A risk of caecal perforation is present, particularly if the diameter is >9 cm.
- *With open ileocaecal valve.* Both large and small bowel distend, the appearances resembling a paralytic ileus.

In equivocal cases, a barium or water-soluble contrast enema can be performed prior to surgery: this locates the site of large bowel obstruction and excludes a pseudoobstruction.

Causes

- *Luminal*: faecal impaction.
- *Bowel wall*:
  - neoplastic: carcinoma;
  - inflammatory: Crohn's disease, ulcerative colitis, diverticular disease;
  - infection: tuberculosis.
- *Extrinsic*:
  - malignant mass, bladder or pelvic malignancy;
  - volvulus;
  - hernia.

Pseudo-obstruction

May be associated with conditions such as pneumonia, infarction and myxoedema. Plain films reveal progressive dilatation of the colon, the appearances resembling mechanical obstruction, and a barium enema may be required to exclude this.

Paralytic ileus

Very common in the postoperative period, due to cessation of intestinal peristaltic activity. Accumulation of gas and fluid contents results in dilatation of both small and large bowel.

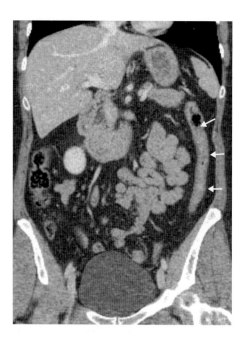

Figure 4.42 Coronal CT reconstruction showing lack of haustration in the descending colon due to ulcerative colitis.

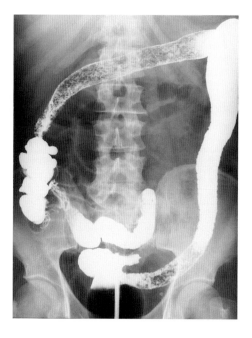

Figure 4.43 Contrast enema: this examination is now rarely used but elegantly demonstrates extensive diffuse mucosal ulceration in the large bowel, with loss of the normal haustral pattern in ulcerative colitis.

Ulcerative colitis

Ulcerative colitis, an inflammatory disease of the large bowel, is characterized by diffuse mucosal damage with ulceration. The inflammatory reaction is limited to the mucosa and submucosa. The aetiology of the disease remains unknown.

Radiological investigations

- Plain abdominal film – may occasionally show an abnormal segment of large bowel, especially when the complication of toxic megacolon arises.
- Colonoscopy is accurate for assessment of the disease.
- CT colonography – replacing barium enema examination.

Radiological features

- Almost always involves the rectum and sigmoid.
- Blurring of the normally sharp mucosal outline.
- Shallow ulceration in continuity from the rectum to a variable distance into the proximal colon, and may involve the whole colon (pancolitis).
- Associated loss of haustral pattern with fibrotic changes may give the bowel a tube-like appearance, the so-called 'lead pipe' colon.

Complications
Colonic

- Toxic megacolon: pronounced bowel distension with an irregular outline, especially of the transverse colon. Barium enema is contraindicated when this complication develops.
- Bowel perforation: in either severe disease or secondary to toxic megacolon.
- Haemorrhage: often profuse.
- Carcinoma: increased incidence especially when there is a pancolitis and the disease has been present for more than 10 years.
- Stricture formation: may be multiple with a smooth outline.

Extracolonic

- Sacroiliitis; arthritis; uveitis; sclerosing cholangitis.

Treatment

- Medical: steroids, systemic and local application in large bowel; sulfasalazine and related drugs.
- Surgical: total proctocolectomy with ileo-anal anastomosis in severe disease with intractable symptoms.

> **Key point**
>
> There is a greater incidence of colonic carcinoma with ulcerative colitis

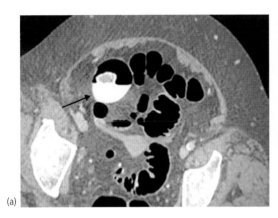
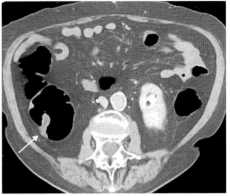

(a) (b)

Figure 4.44 (a, b) CT colonography showing polyps (arrows). A clean colon is essential as faecal residue can have a similar appearance.

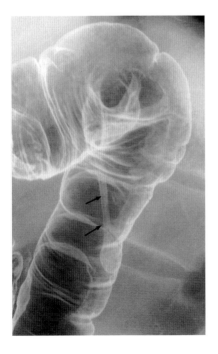

Figure 4.45 Pedunculated colonic polyp (arrows).

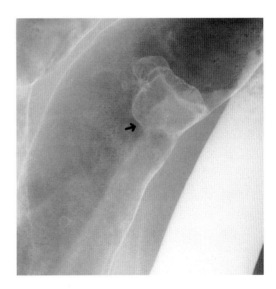

Figure 4.46 Sessile polyp (arrow).

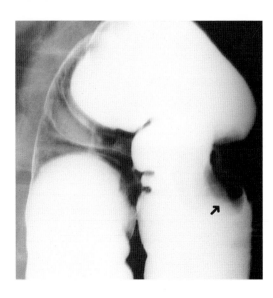

Figure 4.47 Sessile polyp.

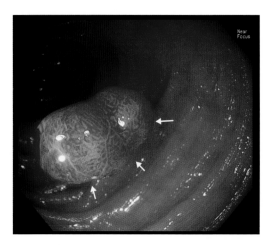

Figure 4.48 Colonoscopy showing a large polyp (arrows).

Colonic polyps

Colonic polyps are localized mass lesions arising from the mucosa of the colon that protrude into the lumen. They may be broad based (sessile) or on a stalk (pedunculated) and can occur anywhere in the colon. The majority of polyps are benign adenomas, especially those with long thin stalks.

Radiological features

- Barium enema – polyps are seen as a filling defect on the barium-filled views, or outlined by barium on the air-filled projections.
- CT colonography – accurate for diagnosis of polyps.
- Colonoscopy.

Complications

Malignancy in a polyp should be considered if there is:

- irregularity at the base or periphery;
- a flat lesion with a broader base than height;
- growth on serial examinations;
- a polyp >10 mm.

Treatment

Small polyps can be snared and removed at colonoscopy; perforation and haemorrhage are infrequent complications of this procedure; larger lesions need formal surgical resection.

Additional features

Multiple polyps may be found in the following.

- Familial adenomatous polyposis: an autosomal-dominant inherited disease with multiple polyps, which become clinically apparent in the second decade. The risk of malignancy developing is almost 100%.
- Peutz–Jeghers syndrome: polyps are hamartomas with no malignant potential.
- Inflammatory bowel disease: in ulcerative colitis, less commonly Crohn's disease, areas of mucosal hyperplasia may be present (pseudopolyps).

Classification

- Neoplastic: adenoma, adenocarcinoma.
- Hamartomatous: Peutz–Jeghers syndrome.
- Inflammatory: Crohn's disease, ulcerative colitis. Hyperplastic overgrowth of regenerating mucosa produces inflammatory pseudopolyps.

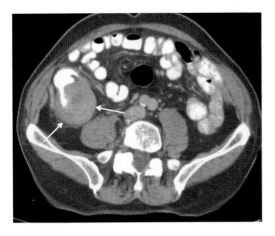

Figure 4.49 CT abdomen: caecal carcinoma (arrows).

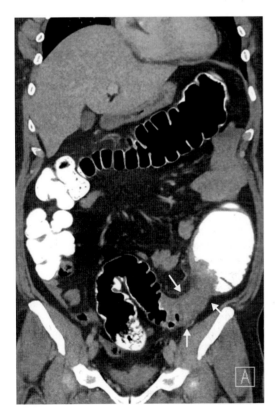

Figure 4.50 Coronal CT showing large mass due to colon carcinoma (arrows).

Colonic carcinoma

Carcinoma of the colon, usually an adenocarcinoma, is the commonest malignancy of the intestinal tract, with the preponderance of lesions occurring in the rectosigmoid region. Predisposing factors include hereditary polyposis syndromes, chronic inflammatory bowel disease, family history of colonic carcinoma and possibly dietary causes.

Radiological investigations

- Chest X-ray.
- Barium enema or colonoscopy.
- CT colonography.
- CT/MRI for staging and preoperative work-up.

Radiological features

Barium enema or CT colonography may demonstrate a malignant polyp. More advanced tumours have the following features.

- Annular carcinoma: predominantly infiltrates the bowel wall circumferentially causing irregular luminal narrowing with an 'apple-core' deformity. Overhanging edges cause a 'shouldering' defect.
- Polypoidal mass: produces an intraluminal filling defect, most commonly in the caecum.

Complications

- Obstruction: sometimes a presenting feature. Plain abdominal films may localize the level of obstruction. In equivocal cases, water-soluble contrast enema readily defines the site of obstruction prior to surgery.
- Perforation: secondary to bowel distension caused by tumour obstruction; may present with peritonitis.
- Fistula formation: from malignant infiltration of adjacent structures.

Differential diagnosis of colonic narrowing

- Diverticular disease: usually in sigmoid colon.
- Crohn's disease: strictures may be single or multiple.

- Ulcerative colitis: benign or malignant strictures develop after prolonged bowel involvement.
- Extrinsic: inflammatory or neoplastic infiltration.
- Radiotherapy.
- Tuberculosis.
- Ischaemia.

> **Key point**
>
> A stricture in the colon must be considered to be malignant unless proved otherwise

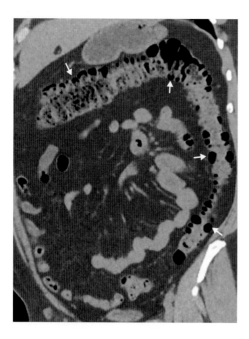

Figure 4.51 Coronal CT reconstruction showing extensive diverticular disease throughout the colon (arrows).

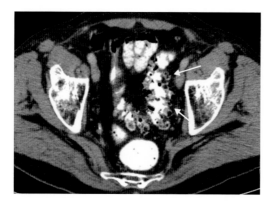

Figure 4.52 CT pelvis: diverticular disease of the sigmoid colon (arrows).

Diverticular disease

Diverticular disease is a common disorder with colonic smooth muscle hypertrophy associated with pouch-like protrusions between the thickened muscle fibres. There is herniation of the mucosa and submucosa through sites of weakness in the bowel wall. The sigmoid is the most frequently affected (>90%), but diverticula may arise from any part of the colon. A low-fibre diet is likely to be an aetiology of this condition.

Radiological investigations

- Barium enema.
- CT colonography.
- Ultrasound, CT and mesenteric angiography for complications.

Radiological features

- Barium enema examination readily demonstrates the outpouchings as smooth, round projections from the bowel wall.
- Diverticula vary considerably in size, from being just visible, to oval or round sacs several centimetres in diameter.
- Barium may persist in the diverticula for several weeks as there is no mechanism for emptying.
- The sigmoid colon may be narrow and irregular, and sometimes the appearances are very difficult to distinguish from a carcinoma.

Complications

- Diverticulitis: inflammatory changes leading to attacks of abdominal pain and fever.
- Pericolic abscess: perforation of a diverticulum often results in a localized pericolic abscess. A barium enema may show a sinus track leading from the sigmoid into the abscess. Ultrasound or CT may demonstrate the localized collection, which can sometimes be drained percutaneously.
- Perforation: free perforation of the diverticulum or abscess into the peritoneal cavity can give rise to a faecal peritonitis.
- Fistula formation: may result from rupture of an abscess or inflamed diverticulum into an adjacent organ, the commonest being the bladder (vesicocolic fistula), with pneumaturia as a presenting symptom. Fistulae may lead into the vagina, ureter, small bowel, colon or skin.
- Haemorrhage: probably from erosion of a bowel wall artery, often from a right-colon diverticulum.

Bleeding can be profuse and mesenteric angiography may localize the exact site of bleeding.

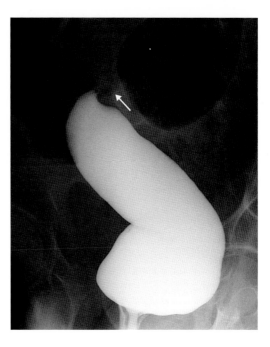

Figure 4.55 Contrast enema demonstrating the typical 'bird's beak' appearance at the site of obstruction in sigmoid volvulus (arrow).

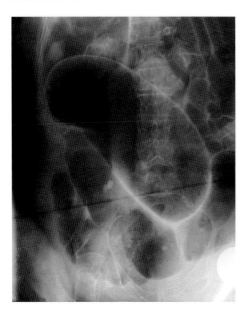

Figure 4.53 Sigmoid volvulus with a grossly distended sigmoid colon.

Volvulus

Volvulus is the twisting of a segment of gut with subsequent obstruction.

Torsion

Torsion refers to twisting without obstruction. The stomach, small bowel, caecum and sigmoid can all be involved, but the sigmoid is the most frequently affected.

Gastric volvulus

Rotation of the stomach occurs in either the vertical or organo-axial plane (line from pylorus to cardia).

Small-bowel volvulus

Mesenteric anomalies with a mobile bowel allow abnormal rotation and twisting, resulting in mechanical obstruction with possible vascular compromise.

Caecal volvulus

The caecum twists on its long axis. The distended gas-filled caecum is characteristically displaced upwards

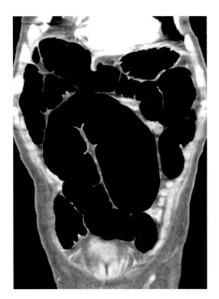

Figure 4.54 Coronal CT showing a distended sigmoid due to a volvulus.

and into the left upper quadrant, with an empty right iliac fossa. The distal colon is devoid of air, and growing caecal dilatation leads to a threat of perforation.

Sigmoid volvulus

Elderly and long-term psychiatric patients are particularly prone to this condition. Sigmoid volvulus occurs when there is rotation of the sigmoid about its axis, especially in a long redundant loop, to give rise to a closed-loop obstruction. Unrelieved obstruction may lead to vascular compromise, bowel infarction or perforation.

Radiological features

The sigmoid loop can become very dilated to occupy the whole of the abdomen. It has the appearance of an inverted U with three dense lines, two lateral walls and a central line produced by the two adjacent inner walls, all converging into the large bowel mesenteric root in the pelvis. A barium enema demonstrates obstruction at the level of the volvulus, with the lumen of the bowel tapering to give a 'bird's beak' appearance.

Treatment

Decompression via a rectal tube through the twisted segment. Recurrence rate is up to 80%, and surgical resection of the redundant loop is often required.

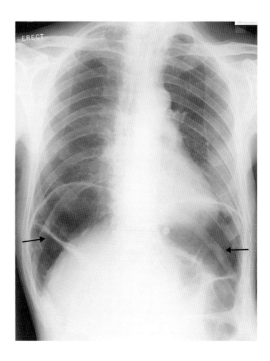

Figure 4.57 Chilaiditi's syndrome: interposition of colon between diaphragm and liver or spleen (arrows).

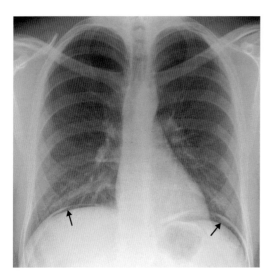

Figure 4.56 Air under the diaphragms (arrows).

Air under the diaphragm

Free abdominal air is also referred to as 'pneumoperitoneum'.

- It accumulates under one or both diaphragms when the patient is erect.
- The erect position has to be maintained for a few minutes before air can be visualized as a crescentic area of lucency between the right diaphragm and liver or left diaphragm and spleen.
- Lateral decubitus abdominal films can be used for very ill patients. The best projection is the left lateral decubitus when free air will be seen between the right lateral margin of the liver and the peritoneal surface.
- Free air will not be seen in up to 20–30% of patients.
- CT is of high accuracy in diagnosing free abdominal air.

Causes

- Post laparotomy or laparoscopy is the commonest cause.
- Viscus perforation (peptic ulcer, colonic diverticulum).

Sometimes difficulty is encountered identifying the free air, either because of viscus distension or confusing gas shadows below the diaphragm. Large bowel interposition between the diaphragm and liver or spleen may simulate free air (Chilaiditi's syndrome).

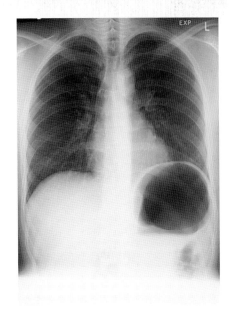

Figure 4.58 Gas distension of the stomach: a common, normal finding.

> **Key point**
>
> Do not mistake Chilaiditi's syndrome for free air under the diaphragm

5

Liver and pancreas

Liver and pancreas: investigations

Plain films

Aids detection of opaque gall bladder calculi, calcification in the gall bladder wall, gas in the biliary tree and pancreatic calcification.

Ultrasound

- Liver ultrasound: visualizes the gall bladder, common bile duct, hepatic and portal veins; an accurate imaging modality for focal or diffuse disease of the liver, detecting secondary deposits, investigation of calculi and jaundice, and as an aid to liver biopsy or interventional procedures.
- Pancreatic ultrasound: useful for suspected pancreatitis or tumour and to assist pancreatic biopsy.

Oral cholecystogram

This investigation is virtually obsolete with the advent of the newer imaging modalities. An iodine-based oral contrast medium is ingested the evening before the examination, with the gall bladder shown as an opacified structure the following day. Calculi are seen as filling defects; a film after a fatty meal shows the extent of gall bladder contraction.

Operative cholangiogram

This investigation is performed at cholecystectomy when the cystic duct is cannulated and contrast injected to outline the common bile duct. Exclusion of common bile duct stones avoids the need for surgical exploration.

T-tube cholangiogram

The study may be carried out after surgery to identify any remaining calculi in the common bile duct. Contrast is injected into the T-tube under fluoroscopic control to exclude residual calculi.

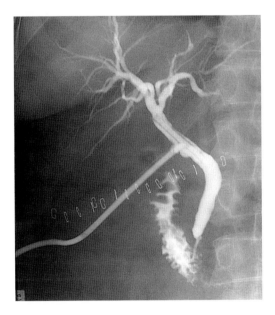

Figure 5.1 Normal T-tube cholangiogram.

Transhepatic cholangiogram

A fine needle is inserted directly into a bile duct in the liver under local anaesthetic. Contrast is injected to visualize the entire biliary system and thus try and elucidate a cause for obstructive jaundice. This technique is used before biliary stenting or to visualize the biliary system when endoscopic retrograde cholangiopancreatography (ERCP) is unsuccessful.

Radiology: Lecture Notes, Fourth Edition. Pradip R. Patel.
© 2020 John Wiley & Sons Ltd. Published 2020 by John Wiley & Sons Ltd.
Companion website: www.wiley.com/go/patel/radiology

ERCP

After the patient is sedated and the pharynx anaesthetized, an endoscope is introduced and advanced through the mouth into the duodenum, with cannulation and contrast injection into the ampulla of Vater, to demonstrate both the bile ducts and the pancreatic duct. Common bile duct stones can be removed through the endoscope by insertion of a catheter with a basket or balloon. Malignant common bile duct strictures can be brushed for cytology assessment and can also be stented.

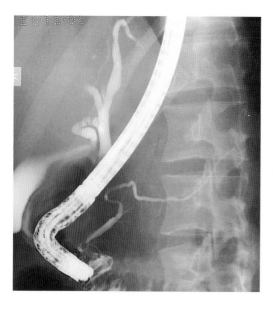

Figure 5.2 Normal ERCP examination showing the pancreatic and common bile ducts.

Isotope scanning (99m-technetium HIDA)

The isotope is accumulated by hepatocytes with excretion in bile. After a short transit time in the liver, the isotope is identified in the gall bladder and bile ducts at 15–20 minutes. Bowel activity is generally seen within an hour of injection. Excretion is severely delayed in biliary obstruction.

Computed tomography (CT)

CT demonstrates the full range of liver and pancreatic disease, including cirrhosis, tumours, pancreatitis and pancreatic carcinoma.

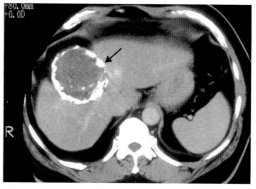

Figure 5.3 CT showing a calcified hydatid cyst in the liver (arrow).

Endoscopic ultrasound (EUS)

EUS assessment of pancreatico-biliary abnormalities is performed in a similar way to ERCP but is less invasive to the ductal system. Unlike ERCP which looks at the ductal system directly, EUS can also look for underlying masses using the adjunct ultrasound and take a fine needle aspirate sample of a lesion. EUS cannot be used to stent the biliary tree.

Magnetic resonance imaging (MRI)

Provides excellent cross-sectional imaging as does CT, but without the radiation. Can either be used independently or as an adjunct to CT for anatomical detail or characterizing hepatobiliary/pancreas abnormalities. For example, bile ducts may be shown without injected contrast by using magnetic resonance cholangiopancreatography (MRCP).

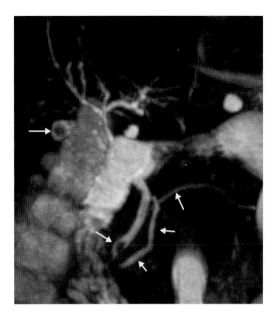

Figure 5.4 MRCP: calculus in the lower common bile duct (arrow) and also in the gall bladder (arrow). Pancreatic duct (arrows).

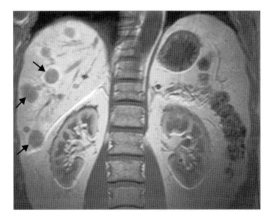

Figure 5.5 MRI: liver metastases (arrows).

Positron emission tomography PET–CT

Providing both functional and anatomical imaging, a tracer (fluorodeoxyglucose, FDG) is injected intravenously and is taken up physiologically but also by metabolically active abnormal tissue. Used in conjunction with a low-resolution CT, it can help identify abnormal areas of tissue uptake. It can be used to stage hepatopancreaticobiliary (HPB) malignancy.

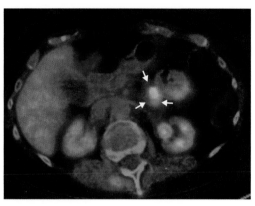

Figure 5.6 PET–CT FDG avid pancreatic body malignancy (arrows).

Angiography

This may be used to identify small islet cell tumours of the pancreas, for preoperative assessment, for the resection of pancreatic tumours and occasionally to identify hypervascular liver tumours; vascular anatomy in portal hypertension may be delineated.

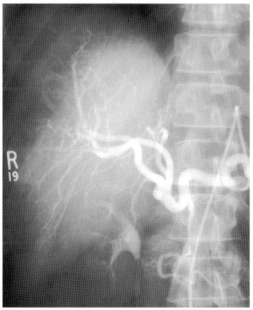

Figure 5.7 Normal hepatic angiogram.

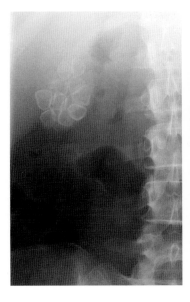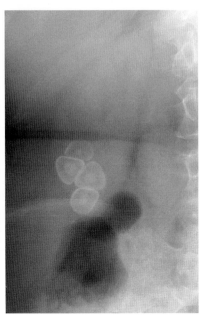

Figure 5.8 Typical appearances of opaque gall bladder calculi on plain films.

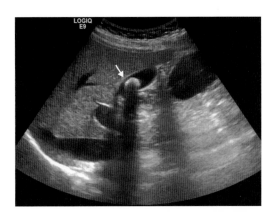

Figure 5.9 Ultrasound of the gall bladder demonstrating a large single calculus (arrow). Note the acoustic shadow posterior to the gallstone.

Gallstones

Gallstones are common and occur in approximately 10% of the population with a female preponderance. There are three main types: mixed, cholesterol and pigment stones. Predisposing causes include obesity, diabetes, Crohn's disease, cirrhosis, pregnancy, infection, haemolytic disease (e.g. sickle cell, thalassaemia) and drugs.

Radiological features

- Plain films visualize approximately 10% of calculi as they are radiopaque. They may be faceted with multiple laminations.
- Ultrasound is the definitive investigation, where gallstones appear as echogenic areas casting a shadow. Gall bladder wall thickening and diameter of the common bile duct can also be assessed. Common bile duct stones are difficult to visualize unless the duct is dilated and can be followed to the ampulla.
- MRCP can also be used to look at the gallbladder and biliary tree for gallstones particularly if the CBD is not well seen on ultrasound.

Complications

- Acute cholecystitis: usually precipitated by obstruction of the cystic duct from a calculus.
- Chronic cholecystitis: chronic inflammation results in thickening and fibrosis of the gall bladder; it is frequently shrunken and non-functioning.
- Biliary tract obstruction: secondary to the passage of a calculus into the common bile duct (choledocholithiasis) with obstructive jaundice.
- Acute pancreatitis: a strong association exists with gallstones. A stone at the lower end of the common bile duct not only impairs pancreatic drainage but also promotes bile reflux into the pancreatic duct.

- Gallstone ileus: occurs when a gallstone ulcerates into the duodenum via a fistula and causes small bowel obstruction by stone impaction.
- Gall bladder carcinoma: rare, but usually associated with gall bladder calculi, chronic cholecystitis, gallbladder calcification and large polyps.
- Empyema: after a gallstone becomes wedged in the cystic duct, there is subsequent distension and inflammation, with purulent material filling the gall bladder.

Treatment

- Cholecystectomy or possible dissolution therapy/ lithotripsy if unfit for surgery.
- ERCP for common bile duct calculi: sphincterotomy with basket or balloon removal of the stone.
- Empyema can be drained percutaneously under ultrasound control.

> **Key point**
>
> Gall bladder calculi are infrequently visible on the plain film and ultrasound is the investigation of choice

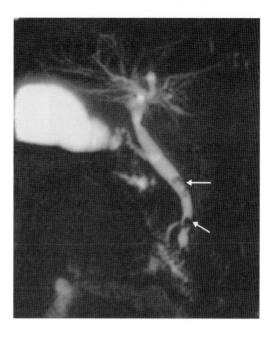

Figure 5.11 MRCP: calculi in the common bile duct (arrows).

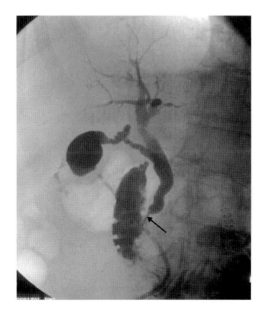

Figure 5.10 Cholangiogram: stricture at the lower end of the common bile duct (arrow).

Common bile duct calculus

The passage of a calculus from the gall bladder into the common bile duct may cause severe pain and often results in obstructive jaundice.

Radiological features

- Ultrasound is the initial investigation of choice and may reveal dilatation of the common bile duct with intrahepatic duct dilatation.
- Calculi in the common bile duct can be difficult to visualize by ultrasound.
- MRCP is usually performed after an ultrasound shows a dilated biliary system unless contraindicated.
- ERCP is a particularly useful investigation, as it will confidently identify calculi as filling defects in a dilated common bile duct, and also offers the capability of removing them, by either the use of a basket or sphincterotomy.
- CT can also be used to look for complicating features of an obstructing calculus.

Additional causes of obstructive jaundice

Benign
- Previous stones/stricture.
- Chronic pancreatitis.
- Iatrogenic.

Malignant
- Cholangiocarcinoma.
- Porta hepatis lymphadenopathy.
- Cholangiocarcinoma.
- Pancreatic and ampullary carcinoma.

Common bile duct stricture

Common bile duct narrowing is caused by numerous disorders resulting in biliary tract obstruction. The presenting features may be pain, jaundice and fever – Charcot's triad.

Radiological features

- Ultrasound is the initial investigation of choice in a patient with jaundice. May demonstrate a dilated common bile duct and intrahepatic duct dilatation.
- CT may demonstrate a tumour mass in the pancreas or liver and will look for disseminated disease.
- MRCP will delineate the biliary anatomy and can identify a pancreas or liver mass.
- ERCP will show luminal abnormalities of the upper gastrointestinal tract in addition to the common bile duct stricture.
- EUS can identify pancreatico-biliary masses and take fine needle aspirates.
- Percutaneous transhepatic cholangiography (PTC) may be required if ERCP is unsuccessful. This may also facilitate positioning of a drain, biliary stent and allow sampling for malignant cells.

Causes

Carcinoma of pancreas; chronic pancreatitis; postoperative; cholangiocarcinoma.

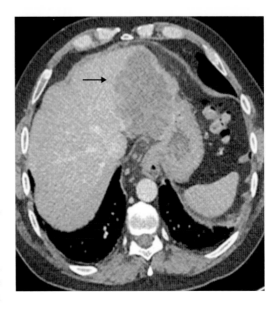

Figure 5.12 CT scan showing a large liver abscess (arrow).

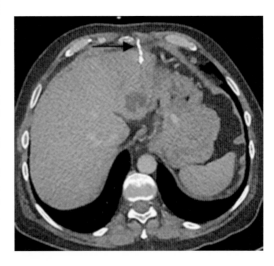

Figure 5.13 CT scan of the abscess after percutaneous drain (arrow).

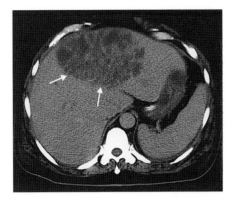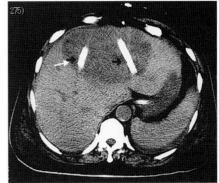

Figure 5.14 Liver abscess: CT scans demonstrating a large low-density lesion in the liver and after percutaneous insertion of drains (arrows).

Liver abscess

A liver abscess is a localized collection of pus often following abdominal sepsis with portal spread to the liver, usually affecting the right lobe of the liver. It is the most common type of abdominal visceral abscess.

Presentation

- Fever.
- Abdominal pain.
- Nausea, weight loss, vomiting.

Causes of liver abscess

- Cryptogenic cause in a large number of cases.
- Biliary tract disease is the most common cause of a pyogenic liver abscess. Biliary obstruction and stagnation may cause bacteria to proliferate. Infections in the portal bed can cause septic emboli to spread to the liver. Liver abscess may also follow suppurative inflammation in the drainage area of the portal vein in portal pyaemia. The latter may arise from inflammatory bowel disease, diverticulitis, appendicitis or a perforated viscus.
- Hematogenous dissemination from septicemia.

Types of liver abscess

- Hydatid cysts (echinococcus) and fungal abscesses are uncommon.

- Amoebic abscesses (Entamoeba histolytica) are common in certain parts of the world. They cannot be readily differentiated from other types of liver abscess.
- In Asia, Klebsiella pneumoniae is an important cause of primary liver abscess.

Differential diagnosis is from cysts which are usually well demarcated in outline with fluid collections, and tumours which appear solid and may contain areas of calcification.

Follow-up resolution of an abscess can be with CT scanning or ultrasound.

Radiological features

Ultrasound may show a single or multiple cavitating lesions. Abscesses are more common in the right lobe and on CT appear as low-density lesions, often showing peripheral rim-like enhancement after intravenous contrast. Occasionally, gas is seen centrally in the liver lesion, confirming the diagnosis of abscess. Hepatomegaly, elevation of the right diaphragm, pleural effusion and lower-lobe atelectasis may all be associated.

Treatment

- Percutaneous aspiration should be performed early for small abscesses under ultrasound or CT control and the contents sent for bacteriology to aid in the diagnosis and start the correct antibiotic therapy.
- Percutaneous catheter drainage may be needed for larger abscesses with an indwelling drainage catheter.

- Surgical drainage when percutaneous drainage fails.
- Antibiotic therapy ideally after specimen analysis from the abscess.

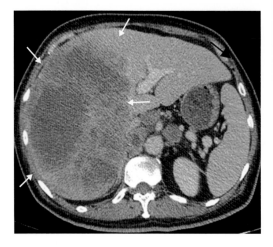

Figure 5.15 Focal mass in the right liver on CT: hepatocellular carcinoma (arrows).

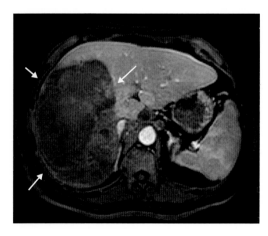

Figure 5.16 Focal mass in the right liver on MRI (same patient as Figure 5.15). The MRI demonstrates better delineation of the lesion and is able to further characterize the mass (arrows).

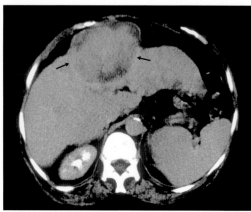

Figure 5.17 CT scan showing a focal mass – hepatocellular carcinoma.

Hepatocellular carcinoma

A common tumour in some parts of the world, but rare in industrialized societies. Risks include Hepatitis B/C carriers, chronic alcohol misuse, biliary cirrhosis, metabolic causes (including haemochromatosis, Wilson's disease, alpha-1 antitrypsin deficiency) and fungal aflatoxin food contamination.

There is an elevated α-fetoprotein in up to 90% of cases.

Presentation

- Surveillance scans in high-risk patients with cirrhosis and Chronic Hepatitis B virus infection.
- Upper abdominal pain.
- Weight loss.
- Fever and deterioration in a patient with cirrhosis.

Radiological features

Multimodality imaging is used which can assess for the three principal types: focal, multinodular or infiltrative. The tumour is assessed for local invasion including the vessels and more disseminated disease.

- Ultrasound is a good first-line investigation to assess the liver for background liver disease and an obvious mass.
- CT evaluates the liver but also looks for ancillary features of chronic liver disease, e.g. splenomegaly, varices and ascites associated with portal hypertension.
- MRI liver with contrast can further characterize suspicious liver lesions seen on CT.

Treatment

Hepatocellular carcinoma is an aggressive tumour with average survival times from six months to two years.

- Liver resection for localized tumours.
- Liver transplantation.
- Ablation therapies, including radiation, microwave and cryogenic.
- Chemotherapy.
- Arterial embolization.

> **Key point**
>
> Hepatocellular carcinoma is the most common primary hepatic tumour and one of the most common cancers worldwide

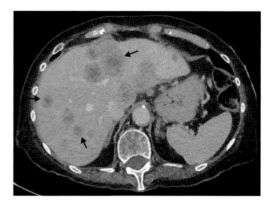

Figure 5.18 CT scan of the liver demonstrating multiple well-defined metastases of different densities (arrows).

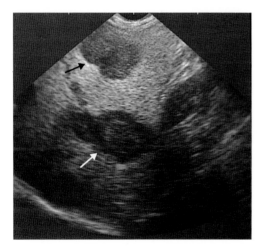

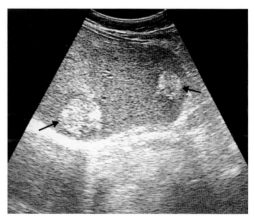

Figure 5.19 Ultrasound of the liver; low- and high-echo metastases (arrows).

Liver metastases

The liver is the most common organ as a site of secondary deposits. The most frequent neoplasms to metastasize to liver are those of colon, stomach, pancreas, breast and lung. Secondary deposits are much more common than primary liver tumours.

Presentation

- Asymptomatic finding.
- Hepatomegaly.
- Ascites.
- Weight loss.
- Abnormal liver enzymes and jaundice.
- Preoperative check prior to surgery for primary carcinoma.
- Follow-up of primary carcinoma.

Radiological investigation

- Plain films.
- Ultrasound.
- CT/MRI.
- Arteriography.
- Percutaneous biopsy (guided by ultrasound or CT).

Radiological features

- Plain films are usually not contributory. They may show hepatomegaly and occasionally calcified liver metastases.
- Ultrasound has a high degree of accuracy and in a good-quality study is a very sensitive examination for the detection of metastases. The normal liver has a smooth outline with a homogeneous echo pattern. The essential feature of ultrasound is to demonstrate an abnormal echo pattern in the liver, metastases often being echo-poor, cystic, hyperechoic or diffusely infiltrative.

- CT and MRI can assess for liver burden of metastases.
- MRI can be more sensitive for smaller liver lesions and for lesion conspicuity.
- Arteriography can facilitate treatment. Chemotherapy/embolization (transarterial chemoembolisation, TACE) may be undertaken directly via the hepatic artery.

Differential diagnosis

Haemangioma (common); hepatoma; abscess; haematoma.

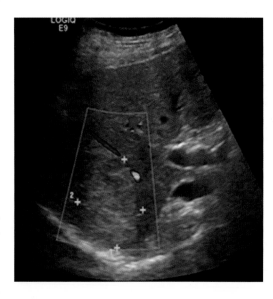

Figure 5.20 Ultrasound liver showing a well-defined echogenic focus consistent with a haemangioma. MRI or CT will further characterize the lesion.

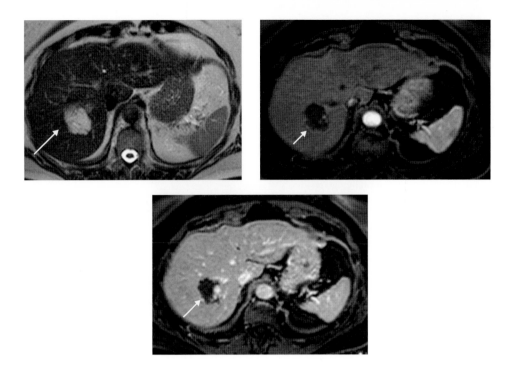

Figure 5.21 MRI T2 sequences arterial and delayed phases characterizing a benign haemangioma (arrow 3).

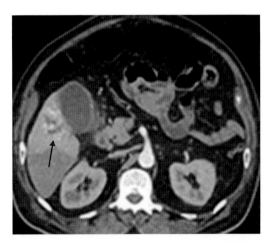

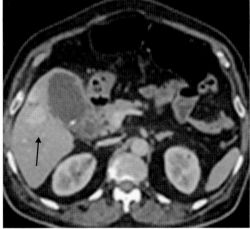

Figure 5.22 CT liver (arterial phase) showing peripheral discontinuous enhancement of the liver haemangioma (arrow).

Figure 5.23 CT liver (portal venous phase same patient) showing gradual filling of the liver haemangioma (arrow).

Benign liver tumours

A focal liver lesion may be benign or malignant. Benign lesions should be differentiated from liver metastases, cholangiocarcinoma or a hepatocellular carcinoma. Investigations of a solid liver lesion require a contrast-enhanced CT. MRI can be obtained for further evaluation.

Benign focal liver lesions include
- Haemangioma, most common benign lesion.
- Regenerative nodules in cirrhosis, composed of regenerating liver tissue.
- Hepatic adenoma, a benign epithelial tumour often associated with oral contraceptive use.
- Focal nodular hyperplasia, most commonly found in young women.

Diagnostic studies
- Ultrasound.
- Contrast-enhanced CT scanning.
- Contrast-enhanced MRI scanning.
- Fine needle biopsy

Diagnostic studies often cannot reliably distinguish between benign tumours except haemangiomas. These are non-malignant vascular liver lesions found typically during imaging for unrelated conditions, but once found, need to be differentiated from a malignant liver lesion. It has a higher prevalence in females than males (5:1). Occasionally, pain and large size can be an indication for surgery.

Presentation

- Asymptomatic incidental finding on imaging.
- When large, complications can occur with pain, bleeding, thrombosis or rupture.

Radiological features

- Ultrasound shows a well-defined echogenic lesion with occasionally showing a feeding vessel.
- CT – Multiphase CT shows typical characteristics with low attenuation on non-contrast scans,

peripheral discontinuous nodular enhancement on arterial scans with gradual filling on the venous and delayed phases.
- MRI low signal T1, high signal T2 and demonstrate similar enhancement to CT.

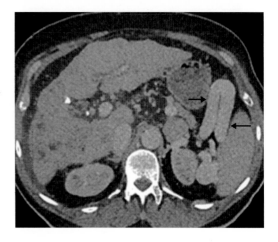

Figure 5.24 Non-contrast CT demonstrating irregular contour liver, and varices (arrows) indicating portal hypertension.

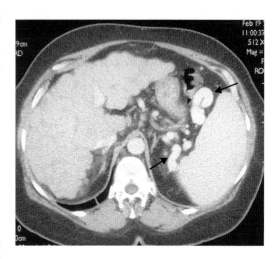

Figure 5.25 CT of upper abdomen: irregular liver in cirrhosis with large varices around the spleen in portal hypertension (arrows).

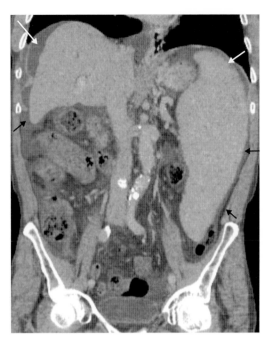

Figure 5.26 Coronal CT showing a large spleen (arrow). Ascitic fluid is seen around the liver (arrow).

Cirrhosis

Represents chronic fibrosis causing a distorted liver architecture. Patients with cirrhosis are at risk of primary liver malignancy.

Causes of cirrhosis

- Alcoholic liver disease.
- Chronic viral disease Hepatitis B, C.
- Other causes such as biliary tract disease (primary sclerosing cholangitis, primary biliary cirrhosis), metabolic (haemachromatosis), autoimmune and drug therapy.

Presentation

- Anorexia, weight loss.
- Jaundice.
- Gastrointestinal haemorrhage: hematemesis, melena.
- Abdominal distension and ascites.
- Hepatic encephalopathy.
- Ascites.
- Hepatomegaly, splenomegaly.

Radiological features

- Plain chest films may feature pleural effusions depending on the severity of decompensation.
- Abdominal film may reveal hepatosplenomegaly.
- Ultrasound and CT scanning show liver parenchymal changes and can assess for features of portal hypertension, portal thrombosis, varices and liver decompensation. There may be hepatosplenomegaly, but the liver may be small and shrunken in the late stages.
- MRI is able to characterize liver lesions with more accuracy in the context of cirrhosis.

Treatment

- Medical treatment.
- Liver biopsy to diagnose cirrhosis.
- Supportive ultrasound guided drainage can be performed for ascites.

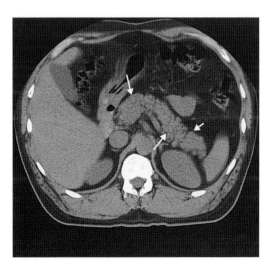

Figure 5.27 CT scan of a normal pancreas (arrows).

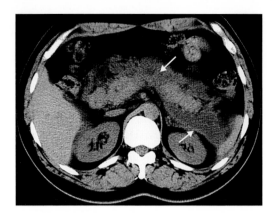

Figure 5.28 Acute pancreas: CT scan showing inflammatory exudate surrounding the pancreas (arrows).

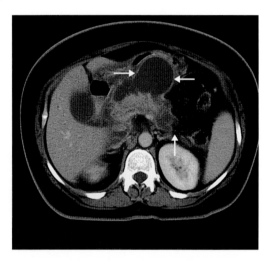

Figure 5.29 CT scan showing a well-defined, low-density pseudocyst (→←). The tail is not enhancing indicating pancreatic necrosis (↑).

Acute pancreatitis

Acute pancreatitis, an inflammatory condition of the pancreas, has many aetiologies, but gallstones and alcohol abuse account for the vast majority. Mumps, certain drugs, surgical trauma and pancreatic carcinoma are some of the precipitating causes. Pancreatic function and morphology usually return to normal after an acute attack.

Radiological features

- *Chest X-ray* – often reveals pleural effusions (high amylase content); more common on the left side.
- *Abdominal film* – may show gallstones, absence of gas in the abdomen or an ileus. A 'sentinel loop of bowel' may be seen in the peripancreatic region.
- Ultrasound may visualize gallstones, dilatation of common bile duct, enlarged pancreas with dilatation of the pancreatic duct.
- CT – accurate in delineating the enlarged oedematous pancreas and its complications, such as necrosis, haemorrhage and fluid collections. Contrast enhancement helps the surgeon by indicating the remaining viable organ. Serial CT follows the evolution of the inflammatory process.

Complications

- Pleural effusions and basal atelectasis.
- Necrotizing pancreatitis: proteolytic destruction of pancreatic parenchyma, with necrosis of the pancreas and surrounding fat, resulting in a solid inflammatory pancreatic mass called a 'phlegmon'. A high mortality rate is to be expected when this complication arises.
- Pancreatic ascites: due to perforation of the pancreatic duct.
- Jaundice from compression of the lower end of the common bile duct by the oedematous pancreas or by common bile duct calculi.
- Abscess: occurs after an acute attack, when a collection of necrotic pancreatic tissue becomes infected.
- Pseudocyst formation: results from escape of pancreatic secretions from the pancreatic duct or exudation from the surface of the inflamed pancreas; the lesser sac is the commonest location.
- Pseudoaneurysm formation: inflammatory weakening of the surrounding arteries may cause a catastrophic haemorrhage.
- Portal/splenic vein thrombosis.
- Hypocalcaemia.
- Hyperglycaemia.

> **Key point**
>
> In severe acute pancreatitis, contrast-enhanced CT scans help determine the presence of pancreatic necrosis and related complications

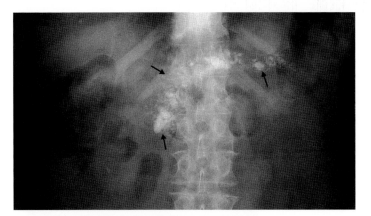

Figure 5.30 Pancreatic calcification on a plain upper abdominal film (arrows).

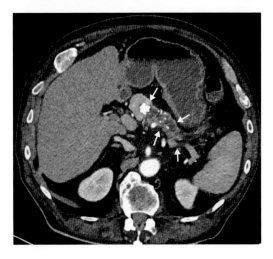

Figure 5.31 CT scan: pancreatic calcification in an atrophic pancreas (arrows).

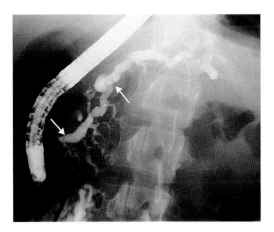

Figure 5.32 ERCP: dilated irregular pancreatic duct in chronic pancreatitis (arrows).

Chronic pancreatitis

Chronic pancreatitis is most commonly caused by alcohol abuse. The basic pathology is ductal stenosis and obstruction resulting in atrophy and fibrosis of the pancreas; irreversible damage to the pancreas results in abnormal pancreatic morphology. Gallstones are frequently associated with chronic pancreatitis.

Presentation

Intermittent abdominal pain; weight loss; diarrhoea; steatorrhoea; jaundice; diabetes.

Radiological features

- Pancreatic calcification on abdominal X-ray or CT is virtually pathognomonic of chronic pancreatitis. Calcification is noted in approximately 50% of cases, CT being more accurate in its detection than a plain abdominal X-ray. Almost all calcification is intraductal, and it may be either diffusely spread or localized to a specific region.
- Ultrasound and CT may show a small, irregular atrophic pancreas with altered parenchymal pattern. Ascites may be associated.
- MRI shows loss of signal intensity on TI sequence, atrophic pancreas and ectatic side branches of the pancreatic duct.
- ERCP with cannulation and injection of contrast into the pancreatic duct may show an irregular dilated duct with stenoses, obstruction and non-filling of the side branches. Pseudocysts may fill if they communicate.

Complications

- Jaundice from bile duct obstruction.
- Pseudocyst formation.
- Splenic, portal or mesenteric vein thrombosis.
- Malabsorption.

Treatment

- Medical: correcting diabetes and malabsorption by diet, insulin and pancreatic supplements.
- Surgical: cholecystectomy for gallstones; intervention for complications such as biliary obstruction or pseudocyst formation; partial or total pancreatectomy with drainage procedure of pancreatic duct. Cysts may be drained into the stomach under radiological guidance.

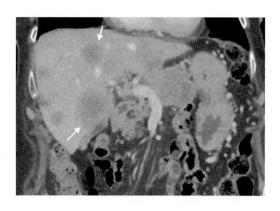

Figure 5.34 CT abdomen (coronal same patient): pancreatic carcinoma showing concurrent liver metastases (arrows).

> **Key point**
>
> Pancreatic calcification is virtually pathognomonic of chronic pancreatitis

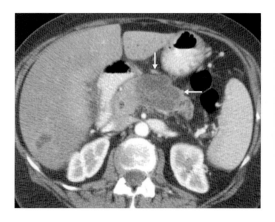

Figure 5.33 CT abdomen (axial): pancreatic carcinoma (arrows).

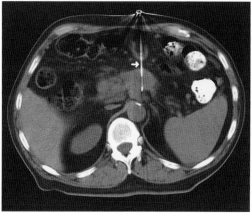

Figure 5.35 Pancreatic biopsy under CT control. The biopsy needle has been inserted directly through the anterior abdominal wall (arrow).

Pancreatic carcinoma

Pancreatic carcinoma is the fourth commonest malignant tumour after lung, colon and breast tumours. The most frequent pathological type arises from the pancreatic duct epithelium (adenocarcinoma). Tumours of the body and tail tend to be larger at the time of presentation. There is a poor five-year survival rate. Neuroendocrine tumours such as insulinoma and glucagonoma are much less aggressive.

Presentation

Clinical symptoms usually occur late and at the time of presentation there is often local invasion of blood vessels or bowel. Only a small percentage of patients have the tumour confined to the pancreas.

- Abdominal pain, sometimes severe and continuous.
- Weight loss, anorexia.
- Obstructive jaundice (Courvoisier's sign – distended palpable gallbladder and painless obstructive jaundice).
- Malabsorption, diarrhoea.
- Diabetes.

Radiological features

- *Ultrasound* may demonstrate pancreatic and bile duct dilatation, a distended gall bladder, focal pancreatic enlargement with a hypoechoic mass, liver metastases or ascites.
- *CT* more accurate at assessing local invasion, lymph node involvement and metastases. A definitive diagnosis can often be obtained by a fine-needle or tru-cut biopsy of the mass.
- *MRI* – enhancing mass of the pancreas and bilary duct delineation.
- *EUS* can be useful to obtain a tissue diagnosis and locally stage the lesion.
- *PET CT* – looks for subtle lesions and metastases not well delineated on conventional CT or MRI.

Treatment

Local extension beyond the confines of the organ, invasion of adjacent structures such as the stomach and secondary deposits in the liver or ascites usually render the tumour inoperable: only 10–15% are suitable for attempted curative resection; palliative surgical procedures for relief of jaundice; stenting via ERCP, or if this is not possible, then percutaneous insertion; pancreaticoduodenectomy (Whipple's operation) for small pancreatic or periampullary lesions.

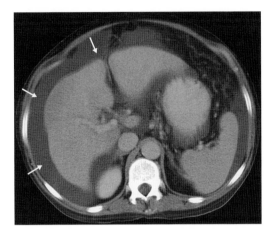

Figure 5.36 Ascites: abdominal CT visualizing ascites as low density (arrows) surrounding the liver and spleen.

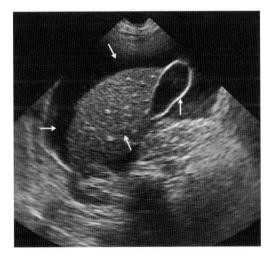

Figure 5.37 Ascites: ultrasound examination demonstrates the free intra-abdominal collection (↘) surrounding the liver (↘) and gall bladder (↑).

Ascites

Ascites refers to an accumulation of fluid within the abdominal cavity; in the supine position, it collects in the most dependent parts, the pelvis and paracolic gutters.

- Haemorrhagic ascites: this suggests malignant involvement of the peritoneum, though it may represent haemorrhage after trauma or liver biopsy.
- Chylous ascites: chyle may rarely accumulate in the peritoneal cavity. Causes include congenital lymphangiectasia, abdominal trauma including surgery with damage to abdominal lymphatic channels, malignant infiltration, filariasis and tuberculosis.

Radiological features

- Plain abdomen films may show generalized haziness of the abdomen, with loss of psoas outlines. Any gas-containing small bowel loops float centrally.
- Ultrasound localizes fluid collections in the abdomen with considerable accuracy. The fluid appears anechoic, is freely mobile and bowel loops may be seen floating in the fluid. It can be aspirated, under ultrasound control, for a diagnostic tap, or percutaneous drainage by means of a catheter can be undertaken.
- CT demonstrates ascites as a low-density margin around the intra-abdominal organs and is most clearly seen adjacent to the liver.

Causes

Transudate

Freely mobile, simple fluid collection.

- Cirrhosis.
- Hypoproteinaemia.
- Renal failure.
- Pericarditis.
- Cardiac failure.
- Budd–Chiari syndrome.

Exudate

Complex fluid collection and may contain solid tissue or inflammatory debris.

- Primary or secondary carcinoma.
- Tuberculous peritonitis.

- Pancreatitis.
- Meigs' syndrome.

> **Key point**
>
> Ultrasound guidance will allow even a small amount of fluid to be aspirated for a diagnostic tap

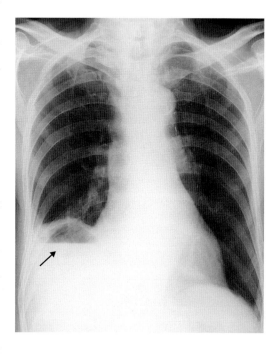

Figure 5.38 Air/fluid level below the right diaphragm in subphrenic abscess (arrow).

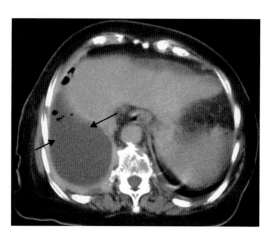

Figure 5.39 CT scan showing subphrenic collection containing air (arrows).

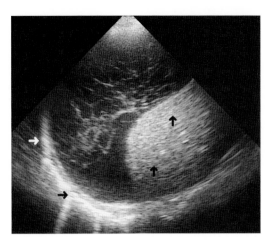

Figure 5.40 Ultrasound reveals the abscess with multiple septations between the diaphragm (→) and liver (↑).

Subphrenic abscess

A subphrenic abscess is a fluid collection between the diaphragm and the liver or spleen. It is a recognized complication of upper abdominal surgery but may occur as a result of perforation of the gastrointestinal tract. The abscess occurs more commonly on the right.

Presentation

Upper abdominal pain; shoulder pain; pyrexia (swinging).

Radiological investigations

- Plain abdomen or chest film.
- Ultrasound.
- CT.
- Isotope scanning.

Radiological features

- Plain chest films may feature a pleural effusion or basal collapse and consolidation. An elevated diaphragm on the affected side and a gas or fluid level under the diaphragm are diagnostic features.
- Ultrasound and CT will demonstrate the volume and extent of the collection.
- Isotope scanning with indium-labelled white cells shows increased activity at the site of the abscess, but is rarely necessary for diagnosis.

Treatment

- Percutaneous drainage under either ultrasound or CT guidance.
- Surgical drainage.

Other sites of abdominal abscess formation

- Psoas abscess: commonly tuberculous but may be pyogenic.
- Pancreatic abscess: follows acute pancreatitis.
- Renal/perinephric abscess: often haematogenous spread or secondary to renal obstruction; diabetics are particularly susceptible.
- Pelvic abscess: results in diarrhoea due to rectal irritation and inflammation.
- Liver abscess: pyogenic or amoebic.
- Appendix abscess: perforation of the appendix may lead to a localized abscess. An abdominal X-ray may show a calcified appendicolith.
- Pericolic abscess: particularly from diverticular disease.
- Intra-abdominal abscess: secondary to bowel perforation.

Urinary tract

The urinary tract: investigations

Plain films

A plain abdominal film can be useful to investigate the urinary tract. This may show: renal calculi, parenchymal calcification, ureteric and bladder calculi, prostatic calcification or sclerotic bone deposits.

Caution should be used in interpreting renal tract calcification as overlying calcified mesenteric lymph nodes and pelvic vein phleboliths are often mistaken for ureteric calculi. Inspiration and expiration films change the position of the kidneys and often confirm that a calcified area in the upper abdomen is a calculus.

Ultrasound

- Ultrasound is one of the most valuable investigations of the urinary tract and the investigation of choice in children.
- It is extremely useful to evaluating renal size, growth, masses, renal obstruction, bladder residual volumes and prostatic size.
- It is inexpensive, does not use ionizing radiation and can be repeated frequently.
- Transrectal ultrasound, where accurate imaging of the prostate is obtained after insertion of the probe in the rectum, is utilized for prostatic biopsy procedures.

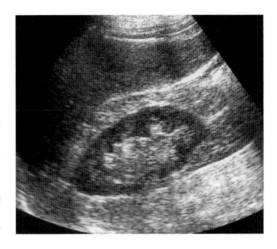

Figure 6.1 Normal renal ultrasound.

Computed tomography (CT)

A low-dose non-contrast CT of the abdomen (CT KUB) is performed specifically to visualize renal and ureteric calculi. Contrast-enhanced CT aids assessment of renal masses, obstruction, retroperitoneal disease, staging of renal and bladder neoplasms, tumour invasion into the renal vein or inferior vena cava (IVC), and evaluation after trauma, surgery or chemotherapy.

Radiology: Lecture Notes, Fourth Edition. Pradip R. Patel.
© 2020 John Wiley & Sons Ltd. Published 2020 by John Wiley & Sons Ltd.
Companion website: www.wiley.com/go/patel/radiology

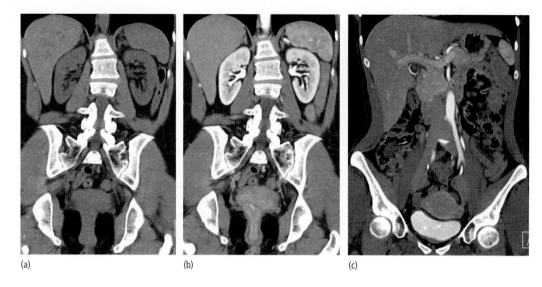

Figure 6.2 (a–c) Urogram showing plain scan (to show calcification) and after contrast both kidneys are excreting with normal calyces and bladder.

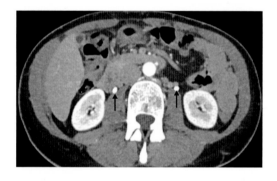

Figure 6.3 Axial scan showing contrast filled ureters (arrows).

Intravenous urography (IVU)

This investigation has now been largely superseded in favour of CT, and is only occasionally used.

Patients with urinary retention and urinary tract infection should initially have an ultrasound rather than an IVU. After an initial plain abdominal film iodinated contrast medium is injected intravenously, images taken at intervals after contrast demonstrate the calyces, ureters and bladder.

Retrograde pyelography

A retrograde pyelogram is occasionally necessary when detail of the pelvicalyceal system and ureter need to be investigated, especially when there is suspicion of an epithelial tumour of the urinary tract. In theatre, a catheter is placed into the ureter after a cystoscopy; contrast injected through the catheter outlines the pelvicalyceal system and ureter.

Percutaneous nephrostomy

This interventional procedure is used to insert a catheter into the kidney for the purpose of relieving an obstructed kidney.

- With the patient in a prone position, a fine-gauge needle is inserted directly into the pelvicalyceal system under local anaesthetic and contrast injected to visualize the calyces, pelvis and ureter.
- This procedure accurately localizes the site of an obstructing lesion, such as a calculus or stricture.
- A nephrostomy provides temporary drainage of an obstructed kidney by percutaneous insertion of a catheter directly into the pelvicalyceal system.

Double J stent insertion

- Following a temporary nephrostomy, a double J ureteric stent can be inserted to leave an indwelling catheter from the renal pelvis to the bladder. The nephrostomy can subsequently be removed.

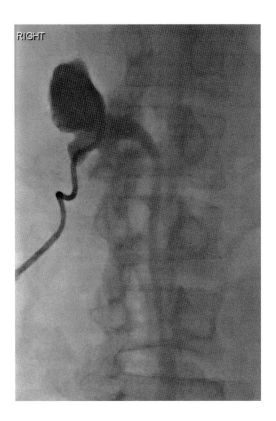

Figure 6.4 Right nephrostomy with a catheter in the pelvicalyceal system.

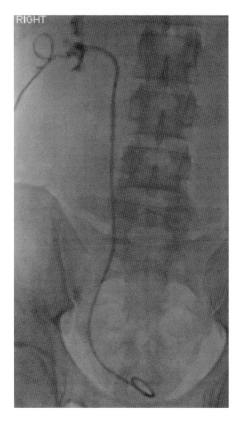

Figure 6.5 An ureteric stent has been inserted following a nephrostomy.

Micturating cystogram

A catheter is inserted in the bladder which is filled to capacity with contrast. After catheter removal, films are taken of the renal tract as the patient is micturating, looking for vesico-ureteric reflux. Careful examination of the urethra in the oblique position is necessary in suspected urethral valves, as they are usually demonstrated only during micturition.

Urethrography

The adult male urethra can be visualized by the following techniques.

- Ascending urethrography: contrast is injected into the meatus and images obtained of the urethra.
- Descending urethrography: after filling the bladder with contrast, the catheter is removed and images of the urethra are taken during micturition. In both studies, the entire urethra must be studied.

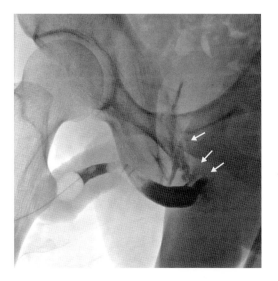

Figure 6.6 Urethrogram showing traumatic injury with complete rupture. There is extravasation of contrast at the site of rupture (arrows).

Nuclear medicine

- Static scanning: technetium-99m DMSA: selective uptake by the renal cells with stagnation in the proximal tubules produces images of the renal parenchyma. The isotope is used to assess function, position, size and scarring of kidneys.
- Dynamic scanning: (1) technetium-99m DTPA: isotope clearance by glomerular filtration produces a dynamic scan, providing information on renal blood flow and renal function. The function of each individual kidney can be assessed, as well as total renal function. (2) Mercaptoacetyltriglycine (MAG3) is preferred in very young children, patients with impaired function and patients with suspected obstruction, due to its superior extraction.

Arteriography

Evaluation of the renal arterial circulation may be necessary for:

- arteriovenous malformation;
- renal artery stenosis;
- anatomical details prior to renal transplantation, or suspected vascular occlusion after surgery;
- further investigation of equivocal renal masses: renal cell carcinomas are usually hyper-vascular with a pathological circulation.

Magnetic resonance imaging (MRI)

Excellent visualization of the adrenals, kidneys and bladder is obtained by MRI, but its principal use is the rapid non-invasive method of imaging the renal arteries.

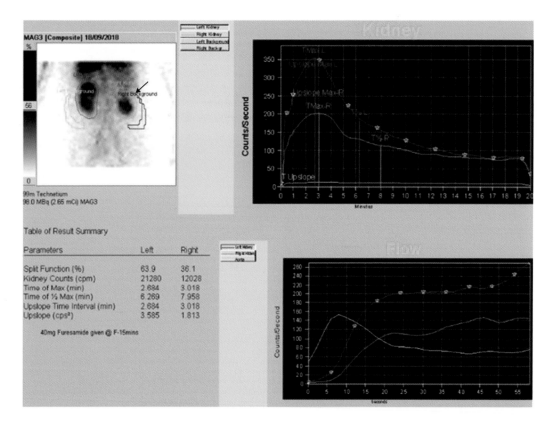

Figure 6.7 MAG3 scan showing significantly reduced function in the right kidney (arrow) due to scarring in the upper pole moiety of a duplex kidney.

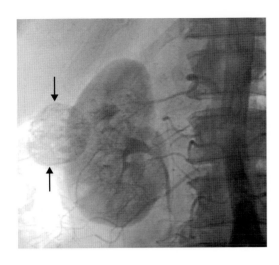

Figure 6.8 Renal angiogram: small right renal cell carcinoma with tumour circulation (arrows).

Congenital renal abnormalities

Unilateral renal agenesis

During urinary tract investigations an incidental absence of a kidney may be discovered. Technetium-99m DMSA isotope scan will confirm this finding.

Renal hypoplasia

The kidney is small but perfectly formed.

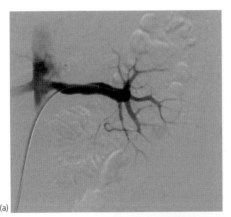

(a)

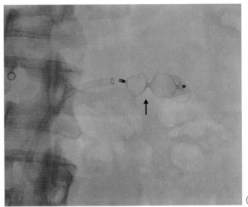

(b)

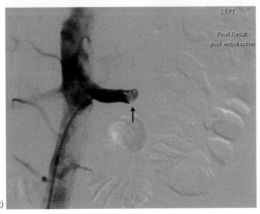

(c)

Figure 6.9 (a) Left renal angiogram prior to renal artery embolization to reduce blood flow to a vascular renal cell carcinoma prior to surgical resection. (b) Large embolization coil in the renal artery (arrow). (c) Post coil insertion showing a completely occluded renal artery (arrow).

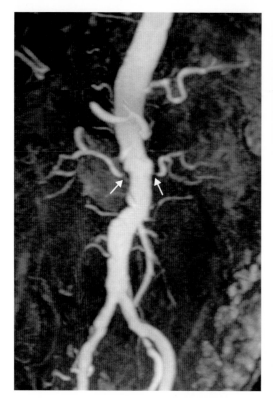

Figure 6.10 MRI: tight bilateral renal artery stenoses (arrows).

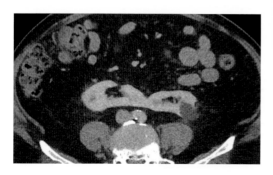

Figure 6.11 Axial CT showing horseshoe kidney.

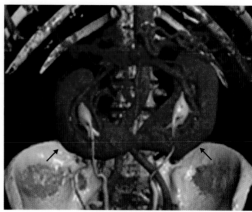

Figure 6.12 Volume render CT scan showing horseshoe kidney (arrows).

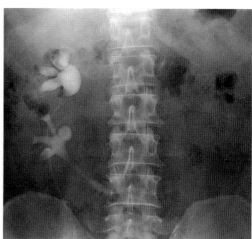

Figure 6.13 Intravenous urography demonstrating crossed fused ectopia.

Crossed fused renal ectopia

One kidney is displaced across the midline and fused to the other normal kidney; ureteric orifices lie in a normal position.

Pelvic kidney

May be associated with vesico-ureteric reflux and hydronephrosis due to an abnormal ureteric insertion.

Horseshoe kidney

Fusion of the opposite renal poles (usually the lower). There is an increased incidence of: pelvi-ureteric junction (PUJ) obstruction; renal calculi; infection.

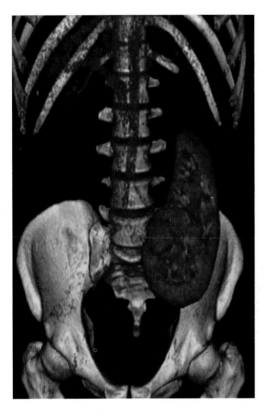

Figure 6.14 Volume rendered CT showing crossed ectopia.

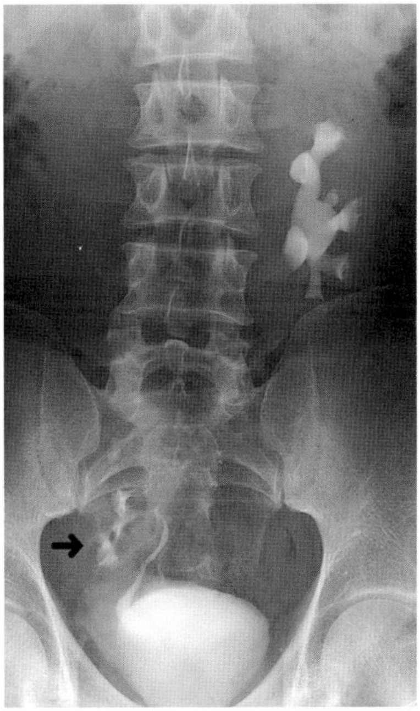

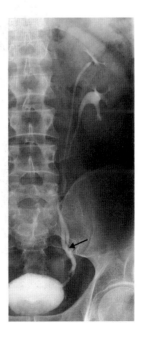

Figure 6.15 IVU showing a pelvic kidney (arrow).

Duplex kidney

The commonest renal anomaly with a variable degree of duplication, ranging from minor changes of the renal pelvis to total duplication of the renal pelvis and ureters.

Polycystic kidneys

Polycystic kidneys are characterized by enlargement of both kidneys with replacement of normal renal tissue by multiple cysts. Expansion and enlargement of cysts compress the renal substance, leading to loss of function and eventually renal failure.

- Polycystic disease of adults – inherited as an autosomal dominant with nearly 100% penetration.
- Polycystic disease of the newborn – discovered in the first few days of life with renal failure and gross enlargement of both kidneys.
- Polycystic disease of childhood – presents at 3–5 years of age with enlarged kidneys and hepatic fibrosis. Death may result from portal hypertension.

Figure 6.16 Left duplex kidney; the ureters join in the pelvis (arrow).

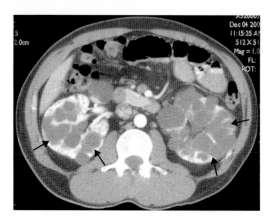

Figure 6.17 CT abdomen: contrast-enhanced scan showing multiple cysts (arrows) in polycystic disease.

Associated features/complications

- Cysts in the liver, pancreas and spleen.
- Increased incidence of intracranial aneurysms. Rarely, polycystic disease may first manifest itself by signs and symptoms of a ruptured intracranial aneurysm (subarachnoid haemorrhage).
- Hypertension.
- Renal calculi.
- Urinary tract infections.
- Uraemia: may eventually need dialysis or renal transplantation.

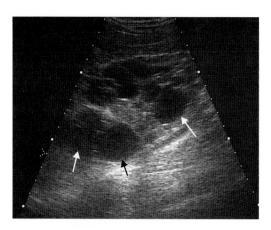

Figure 6.18 Ultrasound: multiple renal cysts seen as low-echo lesions (arrows).

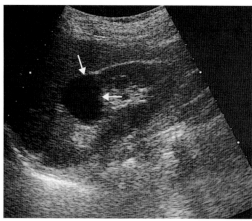

Figure 6.19 Ultrasound: simple renal cyst (arrows).

Presentation

Manifestations of adult polycystic disease usually arise in the third and fourth decades: haematuria; palpable abdominal mass; proteinuria; renal failure.

Radiological features

Renal enlargement is often of massive proportions.

- *Ultrasound and CT* accurately measure the renal size and assess the number and distribution of cysts. The disease may be diagnosed antenatally by ultrasound.
- *IVU* may show elongation, deformity and distortion of the calyces. The renal pelvis may also be deformed by cysts protruding into it.
- *Technetium-99m scanning* will assess renal function.

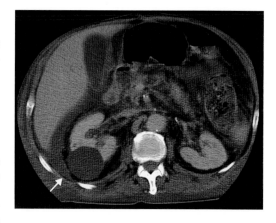

Figure 6.20 CT showing a well-defined right renal cyst (arrow).

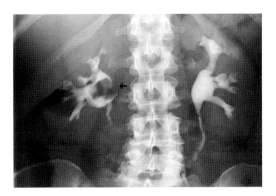

Figure 6.21 Filling defect in the right renal pelvis (arrow), proved to be a transitional cell carcinoma.

Renal cyst

Simple renal cysts are extremely common, occurring with increasing frequency as age progresses. They are often multiple, of varying size and usually an incidental finding. Renal cysts are almost always asymptomatic, of little clinical significance and usually require no further treatment.

Radiological features

- *Ultrasound*: well defined with few or no internal echoes and transmission of the sound beam with posterior acoustic enhancement.
- *Intravenous pyelography*: cysts appear as mass lesions causing a bulge in the renal outline, often with pelvicalyceal distortion.
- *CT*: sharply delineated homogeneous lesions with no enhancement after intravenous contrast.
- *MRI*: well-circumscribed, low-signal lesion (black) or a uniform high-signal (white) depending on the type of sequence used (T1 or T2).

Complicated cysts (haemorrhagic cysts, calcified cysts, cysts with internal septations) need follow-up.

Renal pelvis/ureteric tumours

Tumours arising from the urinary tract epithelium are usually transitional cell carcinomas. They may be polypoidal, plaque-like or form strictures. Squamous cell carcinoma is often associated with either calculi or chronic infection such as schistosomiasis. Haematuria is the main presenting symptom.

Radiological features

- The majority of urothelial tumours produce an intraluminal mass seen on IVU as irregular filling defects, occasionally villous or lobulated.
- Ureteric tumours often exhibit a localized dilatation of the ureter at the site of the tumour, but sometimes antegrade or retrograde pyelography is necessary for further evaluation.
- Ureteroscopy with biopsy will confirm the findings.

Differential diagnosis of filling defect in ureter/renal pelvis

- Calculus.
- Blood clot.
- Tumour.
- Papillary necrosis (diabetes, analgesic abuse).

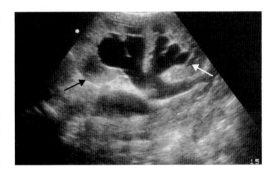

Figure 6.22 Ultrasound: renal obstruction showing dilated calyces (arrows).

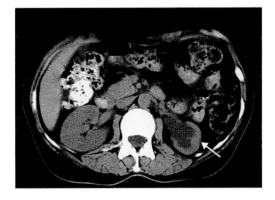

Figure 6.23 CT: chronic left renal obstruction with secondary renal atrophy (arrow).

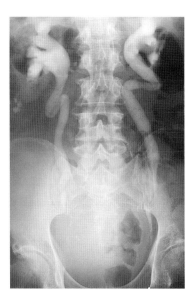

Figure 6.24 IVU showing bilateral dilated calyces and ureters in bladder outlet obstruction.

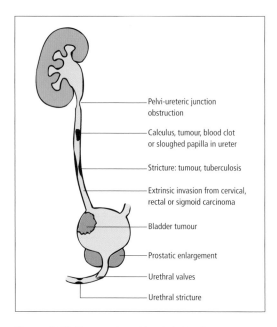

- Pelvi-ureteric junction obstruction
- Calculus, tumour, blood clot or sloughed papilla in ureter
- Stricture: tumour, tuberculosis
- Extrinsic invasion from cervical, rectal or sigmoid carcinoma
- Bladder tumour
- Prostatic enlargement
- Urethral valves
- Urethral stricture

Figure 6.25 Causes of renal tract obstruction.

Renal tract obstruction

Obstruction to the renal tract may occur at many sites: the pelvicalyceal system, ureter, bladder or bladder outlet. The commonest cause is a ureteric calculus, but tumours of the urinary tract or extrinsic ureteric invasion from rectosigmoid or gynaecological tumours are also well-recognized causes. If left untreated, renal atrophic changes may follow.

Radiological features

The different imaging modalities all diagnose renal tract dilatation.

- *Ultrasound*: this is the initial investigation of choice. The distended collecting system is seen as an echo-free area in the centre of the kidney.
- *IVU*: excretion of contrast is delayed with distended and clubbed calyces, often with ureteric dilatation down to the level of obstruction. Slow excretion of contrast may require delayed films up to 24 hours.
- *CT*: demonstrates the distended collecting system and ureters as well as detecting extrinsic causes of obstruction, such as tumours.
- *Isotope scanning*: identifies a slow accumulation and clearance of isotope in the collecting system.

Key point

In a patient with suspected renal obstruction, ultrasound is a rapid diagnostic technique

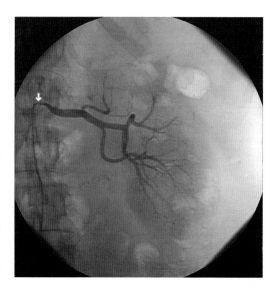

Figure 6.26 Selective left renal arteriogram: stenosis at the origin of the left renal artery (arrow).

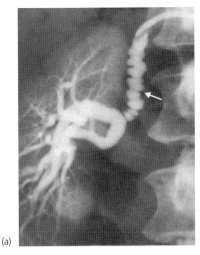 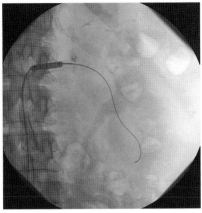

(a)　　　　　　　　　　　　　　　　　　　　　　　(b)

Figure 6.27 (a) Renal angiogram showing a beaded appearance in fibromuscular hyperplasia (arrow); (b) renal artery angioplasty with balloon inflation in the stenosis.

Renal artery stenosis

Renal artery stenosis results from a narrowing of the renal artery, leading to reduction in perfusion pressure, hypertension and a decrease in renal size. It is usually atherosclerotic in nature and may be uni- or bilateral.

Presentation

- Hypertension.
- Deteriorating renal function.

Radiological features

- *Ultrasound* may demonstrate a small kidney. A Doppler examination may show abnormal flow patterns in the renal artery with an increased peak systolic velocity.
- *CT urography* is not reliable and may be entirely normal but classically the affected side shows:
  - delayed appearance and a slow excretion of contrast medium;
  - reduction in pole to pole diameter of >1.5 cm.

- *Isotope scanning* does not accurately diagnose stenosis but may demonstrate a reduced uptake in the affected kidney, with a delay in peak concentration.
- *MRI* is now the investigation of choice for the non-invasive visualization of stenoses.
- *Renal arteriography* is the definitive investigation to show the narrowing, with selective catheterization, and contrast injection into the renal arteries. Stenoses may be due to:
  - Atheroma: commonest cause with stenosis of the proximal artery;
  - fibromuscular hyperplasia: a condition of unknown aetiology, most commonly seen in young women. Irregular intimal hyperplasia gives rise to a beaded appearance with stenosis in the distal renal arteries.

Treatment

- Balloon angioplasty or insertion of metallic stents.
- Surgical reconstruction of the renal artery:
  - vein or prosthetic patch graft;
  - splenic artery revascularization.

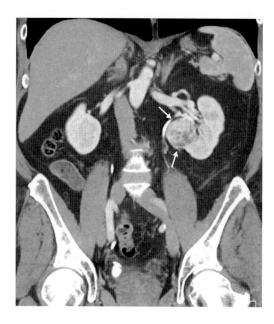

Figure 6.28 Coronal CT demonstrating a renal cell carcinoma (arrows).

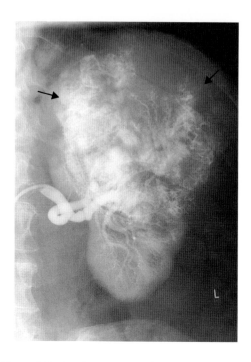

Figure 6.30 Arteriogram demonstrating a pathological circulation in renal carcinoma (arrows).

Wilms' tumour

Wilms' tumour (nephroblastoma) is one of the more common malignancies occurring in children and these may also be bilateral in up to 10% of cases.

Transitional cell carcinoma

Transitional cell carcinomas arise from the epithelium lining the pelvicalyceal system.

Secondary malignant infiltration

Infiltration of the kidneys may be occasionally encountered in lymphoma or leukaemia.

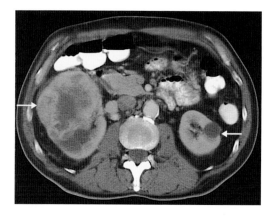

Figure 6.29 Contrast-enhanced CT: large right renal carcinoma (arrow →). Note simple cyst in the left kidney.

Renal tract malignancy

Renal carcinoma

Renal carcinoma arises from the renal tubular epithelium, an adenocarcinoma (hypernephroma); up to 10% may be bilateral.

Presentation

Pyrexia; haematuria; polycythaemia; first symptoms from secondary deposits to lung, bone, liver or brain such as haemoptysis, cough or pathological fractures; left varicocele if the left renal vein is occluded by tumour.

Radiological investigation

Numerous investigations are available including: plain films; IVU; ultrasound; CT; MRI; arteriography and isotope bone scan (for secondary deposits).

Radiological features

- *Plain films*: occasionally show fine stippled or even curvilinear calcification in the renal mass.
- *IVU*: may reveal a soft-tissue mass causing a bulge in the renal outline, an enlargement of the kidney or pelvicalyceal distortion and irregularity. A large tumour may give rise to a completely non-functioning kidney.
- *Ultrasound*: highly accurate in distinguishing between a solid carcinoma and a benign cyst. Blood flow characteristics of the renal tumour can be ascertained and in doubtful cases, a biopsy taken under ultrasound control.
- *CT/MRI*: useful for staging to determine calcification, size and density of the mass; perinephric tissue invasion; invasion into the renal veins and IVC; lymph node enlargement.
- *Arteriography* is not often indicated, but when utilized may demonstrate a pathological circulation in the vast majority of carcinomas.

Differential diagnosis of renal mass

- Cystic with benign features: renal cysts, abscesses, haematoma.
- Solid with benign features: angiomyolipoma, adenoma, haemangioma, papilloma.

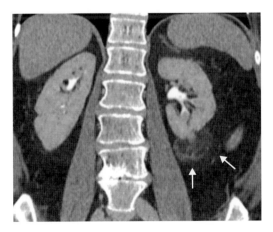

Figure 6.31 CT showing an angiomyolipoma arising from the lower pole of the left kidney (arrows).

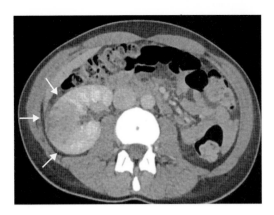

Figure 6.32 CT scan showing area of pyelonephritis in right kidney (arrows).

- Solid with malignant features: renal cell carcinoma, transitional cell carcinoma, Wilms' tumour (nephroblastoma).

Renal angiomyolipoma

Renal angiomyolipomas (AMLs) are the most common benign solid renal tumour and the most common fat-containing tumour of the kidneys. The majority of AMLs are sporadic and the rest are seen in association with phakomatoses such as tuberous sclerosis. Most are detected incidentally on abdominal imaging for other reasons or as part of screening in patients with tuberous sclerosis. AMLs can present with spontaneous haemorrhage, the risk increasing with size (>4 cm).

Radiological features

- Ultrasound: hyperechoic lesions in the renal cortex; may be multiple in the setting of tuberous sclerosis.
- CT/MRI: detection of intralesional fat on CT or MRI is highly suggestive of AML. However, some are fat-poor and a few renal cell carcinoma may also contain fat.

Pyelonephritis

Pyelonephritis is a bacterial infection of the renal pelvis and parenchyma. The infection either migrates to the upper renal tract from the bladder or is seeded haematogenously. The most common infectious organism is *Escherichia coli*. Other implicated organisms include Klebsiella, Proteus and Pseudomonas.

Radiological features

- Ultrasound: often normal, but abnormalities seen include loss of corticomedullary differentiation, oedema (hypoechoic) or haemorrhage (hyperechoic). Ultrasound can detect local complications such as hydronephrosis, abscess formation and perinephric collections.
- CT: unenhanced CT can identify renal enlargement, inflammatory masses, gas or stones within the renal collecting system and obstruction. Contrast-enhanced CT typically shows focal wedge-shaped areas of swelling and reduced enhancement compared with the normal kidney. Perinephric stranding may be present although this is nonspecific.
- MRI: useful in cases when exposure to radiation should be avoided (e.g. pregnant patients). MR imaging findings are similar to those of CT. Affected areas appear hypointense on T1 and hyperintense on T2 compared to normal renal parenchyma.

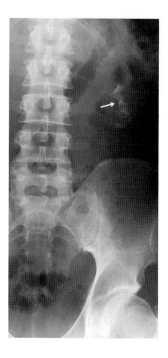

Figure 6.34 Tuberculosis: plain film showing coarse calcification in the lower pole of the left kidney (arrow).

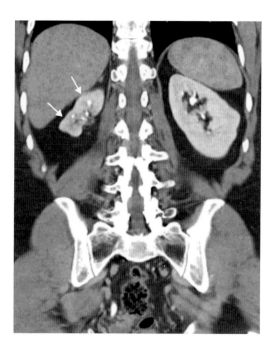

Figure 6.33 Chronic pyelonephritis may result in a small poorly functioning kidney (arrows).

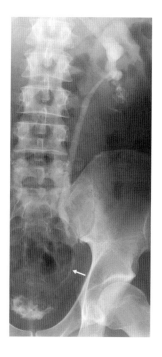

Figure 6.35 IVU showing calyceal and ureteric dilatation due to a lower ureteric stricture (arrow).

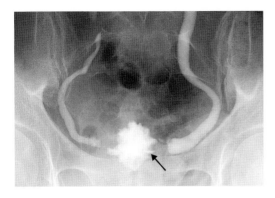

Figure 6.36 Contracted bladder in tuberculosis (arrow).

Tuberculosis of the urinary tract

After pulmonary tuberculosis, the renal tract is the most common site of infection, usually due to haematogenous spread either from pulmonary or bone tuberculosis. Any part of the renal tract may be involved: kidneys, ureters, bladder, seminal vesicles and epididymis.

Radiological features

A chest film should be performed to exclude pulmonary tuberculosis. Plain abdominal films may reveal calcification in the kidneys, seminal vesicles or vas deferens. Calcification is of a variable intensity, ranging from a few small flecks to heavy, dense areas in advanced cases. Gross renal disorganization may lead to a non-functioning kidney (tuberculous autonephrectomy). Testicular ultrasound is useful to delineate epididymitis.

On CT urography, the following features may be found.

- Kidneys: deformities of calyces, strictures, irregular cavity formation and scarring of renal parenchyma.
- Ureters: strictures and areas of narrowing in the ureters, the strictures often being multiple.
- Bladder: tuberculous cystitis – initially there is mucosal oedema but subsequently bladder irregularity with contraction. The bladder has a thickened wall, is shrunken and of a small capacity.

Unilateral non-visualized kidney

Single kidney

May be diagnosed after ultrasound, CT or isotope scanning.

Figure 6.37 Manifestations of renal tract tuberculosis.

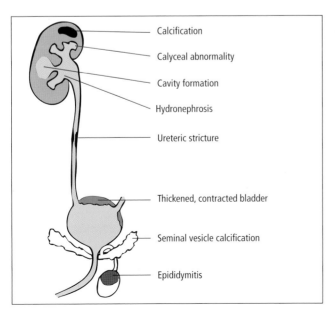

Calcification

Calyceal abnormality

Cavity formation

Hydronephrosis

Ureteric stricture

Thickened, contracted bladder

Seminal vesicle calcification

Epididymitis

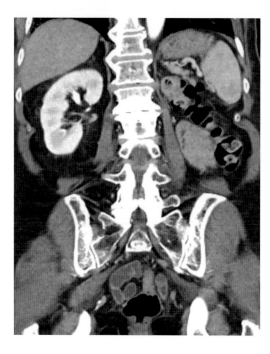

Figure 6.38 Coronal CT: non-visualization of the left kidney.

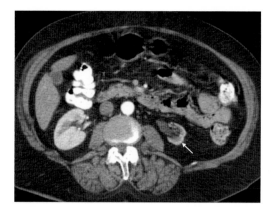

Figure 6.39 CT abdomen; small shrunken left kidney (arrow).

Causes of non-visualized kidney

- Chronic obstruction: ureteric obstruction from calculus, tumour or extrinsic invasion will lead to deterioration of function and atrophy.
- Vascular causes: renal artery occlusion either from severe atheromatous disease or following trauma; renal vein thrombosis.

- Tumour: renal carcinoma infiltrating the whole kidney.
- Chronic infection: chronic pyelonephritis, tuberculosis.
- Postnephrectomy.
- Renal agenesis.
- Ectopic kidney.

Unilateral small kidney

The normal kidney measures 9–14 cm in length, the left usually being larger than the right. However, a difference in size of >1.5 cm is regarded as significant.

Causes

- Chronic pyelonephritis: reduction in renal size, irregularity of outline due to focal areas of scarring and calyceal deformity. Scarring is most common in the upper pole of the kidney over the dilated calyces.
- Ischaemia: renal artery stenosis leading to decreased perfusion.
- Postobstructive atrophy: smooth outline, uniform loss of renal substance, with some dilatation of calyces. Severe obstruction, regardless of the cause, lasting longer than a few days may lead to irreversible loss of renal parenchyma and function, hence the importance of diagnosing and relieving renal tract obstruction.
- Congenital hypoplasia: a small kidney with a smooth outline and a normal pelvicalyceal system.
- Renal infarction: here the scar is opposite a normal calyx.

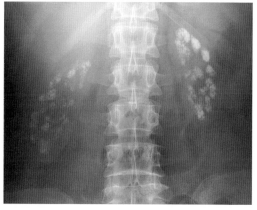

Figure 6.40 Nephrocalcinosis: organized diffuse renal parenchymal calcification.

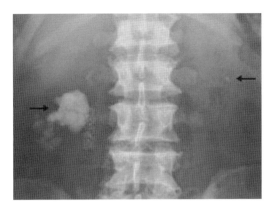

Figure 6.41 Right staghorn calculus (→) and a small calculus in the left kidney (←).

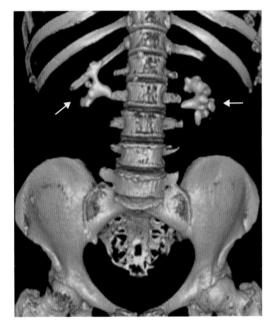

Figure 6.42 Volume rendered CT scan showing bilateral staghorn calculi (arrows).

Nephrocalcinosis

Nephrocalcinosis refers to calcium deposition in the renal parenchyma, either in the cortex or medulla. The calcification is fairly uniform and may be a consequence of the following.

- Hypercalcaemia or hypercalciuria: – hyperparathyroidism, usually primary; renal tubular acidosis;
  - sarcoidosis; multiple myeloma.
- Structural renal abnormality:
  - medullary sponge kidney – congenitally dilated tubules with deposition of calcium; papillary necrosis.

Focal renal parenchymal calcification

- Tuberculosis: variable distribution of the renal calcification.
- Tumours: renal cell carcinoma.

Renal calculus

The majority of renal calculi are pure oxalate, calcium oxalate, calcium oxalate with phosphate, uric acid or cystine. There are several predisposing factors.

- *Stasis* due to congenital abnormalities (horseshoe kidney), pelvi-ureteric junction obstruction, renal-tract obstruction and ureterocoele.
- *Metabolic causes*: hyperparathyroidism; hypercalciuria; uric acid stones after cytotoxic therapy, gout, polycythaemia or after cytotoxic therapy; cystine stones in cystinuria.
- *Infection*: typically *Proteus* infection, often resulting in staghorn calculi.

Radiological features

- A plain abdominal film will generally reveal calculi as they are radiopaque, except for uric acid stones which are radiolucent.
- The majority of calculi form in the calyces and may be seen on IVU as a filling defect in the contrast column.
- Staghorn calculi develop in the pelvicalyceal system and are usually easily visualized on plain films or unenhanced CT.

Treatment

- Extracorporeal lithotripsy (EL).
- Percutaneous removal under radiological control (nephrolithotomy).
- Surgery for large staghorn calculi or when EL and the percutaneous approach have failed.

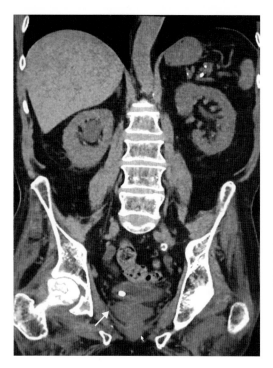

Figure 6.43 Right ureteric calculus at the vesico-ureteric junction (arrow) causing renal obstruction (arrow).

Ureteric calculus

A ureteric calculus tends to be small, often 2–3 mm in diameter, and originates from the kidney. Its progress down the ureter may cause severe abdominal pain; it commonly impacts at the vesico-ureteric junction.

Radiological features

- A plain abdominal film may identify a small area of calcification in line with the ureter.
- Ultrasound may show a dilated upper urinary tract – this is strong indirect evidence of a ureteric calculus.
- An unenhanced CT, without contrast, is a rapid and accurate method of detecting a ureteric calculus.
- An intravenous urogram may be performed to confirm that an opacity is a ureteric calculus, usually identified as a filling defect in the contrast-filled ureter. If causing obstruction, there may be a delay in excretion of contrast, with a variable degree of pelvicalyceal distension and ureteric dilatation to the level of the calculus.

- Nephrostomy or a double J ureteric stent may be needed in severe obstruction.

Treatment

- The majority of calculi <5 mm in diameter pass spontaneously.
- Ureteric calculi can be removed by ureteroscopy or considered for lithotripsy.
- Large calculi: may need open ureterotomy.

> **Key point**
>
> Renal calculi, except uric acid and xanthine calculi, are opaque on plain films

Bladder calculus

Causes

- Descend from the kidney into the bladder.
- Urine infection, especially *Proteus*.
- Urine stasis due to bladder outlet obstruction, bladder diverticulum or neuropathic bladder.
- Foreign bodies in the bladder.

Radiological features

- Calculi may be missed on plain films due to overlying bony structures, gas and faecal shadowing in the rectum, phleboliths or arterial calcification.
- When the bladder is filled with contrast, either at IVU or cystography, bladder stones may appear as filling defects.
- Ultrasound can also detect calculi as echogenic structures casting an acoustic shadow.

Treatment

- Endoscopic removal with lithotrite.
- Large calculi may need open removal.
- EL not widely used for bladder calculi.

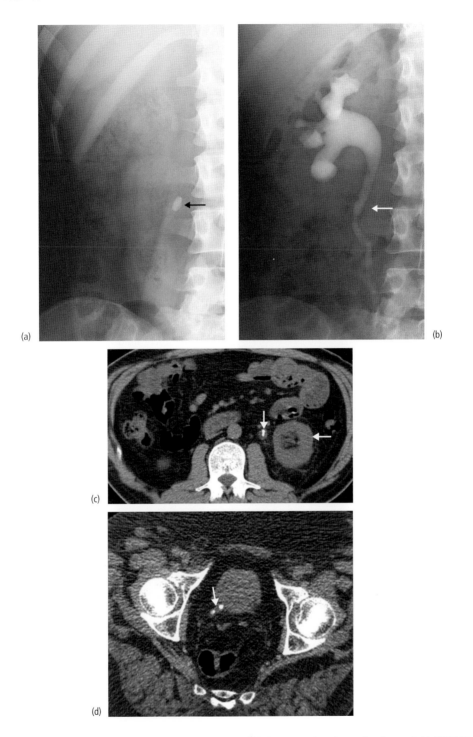

(a)

(b)

(c)

(d)

Figure 6.44 Ureteric calculus: (a) plain film; (b) plain film after IVU demonstrating obstruction (arrows); (c) CT KUB: calculus in the ureter (left arrow); left kidney (right arrow); (d) CT KUB: ureteric calculi near the vesico-ureteric junction (arrow).

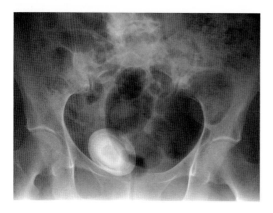

Figure 6.45 Large opaque, laminated bladder calculus.

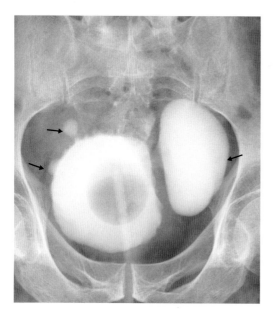

Figure 6.46 Cystogram demonstrating a large left bladder diverticulum (←) with further smaller diverticula on the right (→). An inflated balloon catheter is present in the bladder.

Bladder diverticulum

A mucosal outpouching from the bladder muscle wall results in a bladder diverticulum. They may be:

- acquired secondary to lower urinary tract obstruction or bladder instability;
- associated with a neurogenic bladder;
- congenital.

In males, the commonest cause of diverticula formation is a consequence of raised intravesical pressure with detrusor hypertrophy or from obstruction secondary to prostatic enlargement. Diverticula may be multiple and of a variable size, with some reaching enormous proportions.

IVU, ultrasound and CT

These will all demonstrate diverticula, seen as outpouchings from the bladder wall.

Micturating cystography

Visualizes diverticula, especially during micturition when the outpouchings distend; subsequent emptying of the diverticulum into the bladder at the end of micturition leaves a residual volume and may result in double micturition. Stasis leads to an increased incidence of calculus formation, urinary tract infection and tumour. Residual urine volume in the bladder and diverticulum may be accurately measured by ultrasound.

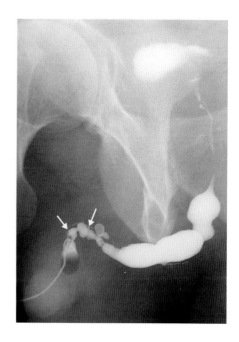

Figure 6.47 Urethrogram: multiple strictures in the anterior urethra (arrows).

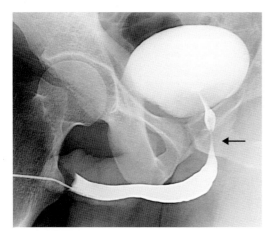

Figure 6.48 Normal urethrogram. The smooth narrowing in the posterior and prostatic urethra (arrow) is normal.

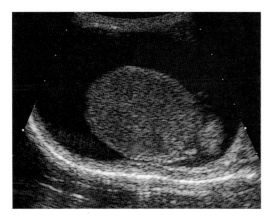

Figure 6.49 Ultrasound: hydrocoele, an occasional manifestation of testicular tumour.

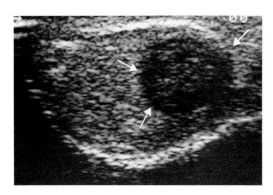

Figure 6.50 Ultrasound: localized altered echo pattern in testicular tumour (arrows).

Urethral stricture

Strictures in the urethra are demonstrated by either a retrograde injection of contrast into the meatus (ascending urethrogram) or after instilling contrast into the bladder, obtaining images as the patient is micturating (descending urethrogram). Strictures present with symptoms of a slow urinary stream and outflow obstruction.

Causes

- Post trauma: following previous instrumentation, catheterization or external trauma. The strictures most commonly occur at the penoscrotal junction or the proximal penile urethra. Straddle injuries compress the urethra against the symphysis pubis with possible rupture; therefore, it is important to perform urethrography before attempting catheterization. A suprapubic catheter is the preferred option in this situation.
- Inflammation: usually occurs in the anterior urethra, often from gonorrhoea, tuberculosis or nonspecific urethritis.
- Neoplasia: develop as a result of malignant infiltration, but is rare.

Testicular carcinoma

Ultrasound is extremely effective in the evaluation of the normal testis and in recognizing a focal lesion; masses of only a few millimetres in diameter are accurately visualized. Ultrasound will rapidly distinguish between an epididymal cyst, a hydrocoele and a testicular tumour.

- Seminoma: these comprise the majority of testicular tumours and appear as homogeneous, well-defined, low-echo mass lesions, sharply demarcated from normal testicular tissue.
- Teratoma: these have a mixed echo pattern and may be cystic or solid. The peak incidence of testicular tumours is between the ages of 25 and 35, with an increased risk in undescended testes. In the older age group, a testicular mass is more likely to be metastatic, rather than a primary tumour. Tumour staging requires a CT thorax, abdomen and pelvis.

> **Key point**
>
> The commonest cause of a generalized scrotal swelling is a hydrocoele and a localized one an epididymal cyst

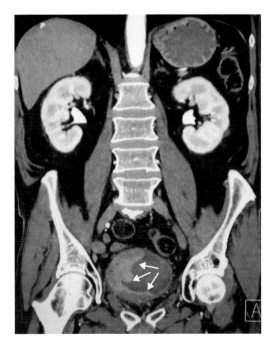

Figure 6.51 Coronal CT reconstruction showing carcinoma of the bladder (arrows).

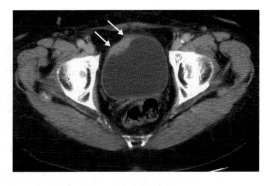

Figure 6.52 CT of the pelvis showing bladder carcinoma (arrows).

Bladder carcinoma

After prostatic carcinoma, the bladder is the commonest site of neoplastic involvement in the urinary tract.

The tumour is usually a transitional cell carcinoma. Predisposing causes include:

- cigarette smoking;
- industrial exposure to aromatic amines;
- chronic infection with *Schistosoma haematobium* (squamous cell carcinoma);
- chronic inflammatory changes due to calculi (squamous cell carcinoma).

Radiological features

- *Cystoscopy* is mandatory in any patient suffering from haematuria.
- *Ultrasonography* is commonly used to assess the upper tracts. However, urothelial tumours of the upper tract are easily missed.
- *CT* or *MRI* is useful in preoperative assessment of intramural and extramural spread, local invasion, lymph node enlargement, and liver or lung secondary deposits. CT urography will assess the renal tract and is superior to the standard IVU.
- *IVU* may be performed to assess the upper urinary tract with respect to:
  - degree of obstruction;
  - state of the ureters;
  - identifying other lesions as transitional cell carcinoma is often multifocal.

Dilatation of the upper tracts usually signifies muscular involvement near the ureteric orifice.

Demonstration of bladder carcinoma on contrast examinations is either by a filling defect in the bladder or an irregular mucosal pattern on the postmicturition bladder films.

Treatment

Treatment depends on the staging of the tumour.

- Superficial tumours: Ta or T1 can be successfully resected endoscopically.
- Invasion of bladder muscle: T2, T3a, T3b may be treated by endoscopic resection, partial or total cystectomy with radiotherapy or chemotherapy.
- Invasion of surrounding organs: T4 into prostate, uterus, etc., need palliative radiotherapy or chemotherapy, or palliative cystectomy with urinary diversion.

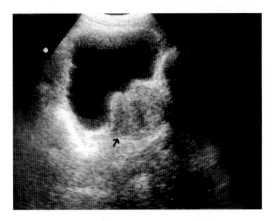

Figure 6.53 Transabdominal ultrasound visualizing the prostate gland (arrow). Transrectal scanning is more accurate.

Prostate carcinoma

Prostatic carcinoma is the most commonly diagnosed cancer in males. The most important prognostic factors for prostate carcinoma include the Gleason grade, the extent of tumour volume and the presence of capsular penetration. High-grade prostate cancer, particularly Gleason grades 4 and 5, is associated with adverse findings and disease progression.

Radiological features

- *Plain films* – sclerotic secondary deposits from primary prostatic carcinoma may be visualized on a plain abdominal film.
- *IVU* – may show a large filling defect at the bladder base, residual urine, the presence of obstructive changes and bladder wall thickening.

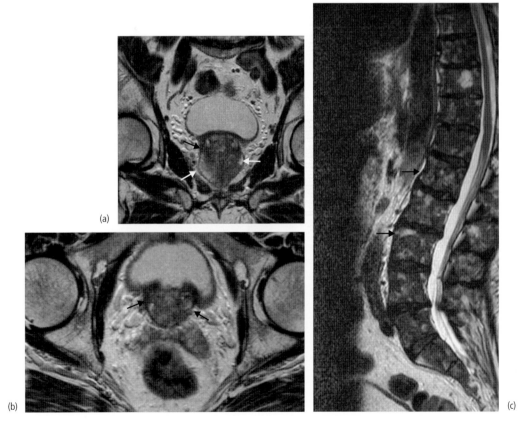

(a)

(b)

(c)

Figure 6.54 (a) MRI – coronal section showing prostate cancer (arrows) as low signal on the T2 sequence; (b) MRI – axial section showing prostatic carcinoma (arrows); (c) MRI – lumbar spine showing extensive metastases (focal areas of high signal shown as white areas).

- *Transabdominal ultrasound* – assesses upper urinary tract and is more accurate than IVU for residual urine.
- *Transrectal prostatic ultrasound* – the scan is performed after the introduction of the transducer into the rectum to assess the size and presence of localized masses. Carcinomas are commonest in the periphery of the gland where they are seen as a focal nodule or diffuse infiltration. Biopsies from various parts of the gland are taken under ultrasound control.

- *CT/MRI* – evaluates tumour spread beyond the prostatic capsule and tumour invasion into the bladder or rectum, with MRI the more precise technique. Patients with a history of prostate cancer who present to the emergency department with sudden onset of weakness of the legs should raise the suspicion of spinal cord compression, necessitating urgent MRI scans with a view to spinal cord decompression.
- *Isotope bone scan* – may demonstrate secondary deposits.

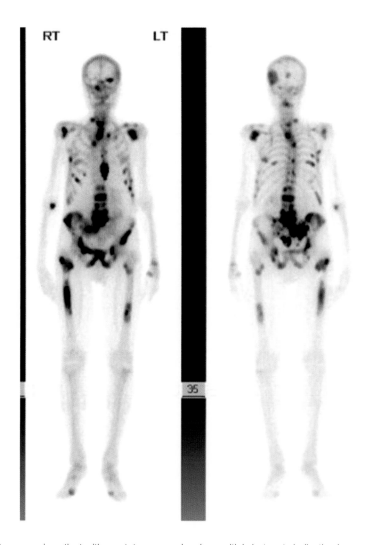

Figure 6.55 Bone scan in patient with prostate cancer showing multiple hotspots indicating bone metastases.

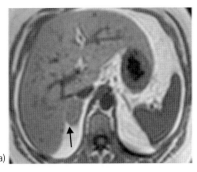
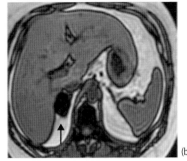

(a) (b)

Figure 6.56 (a) MRI scan showing right adrenal mass demonstrating signal dropout between in-phase imaging (left) and (b) out-of-phase imaging (right), in keeping with an adenoma.

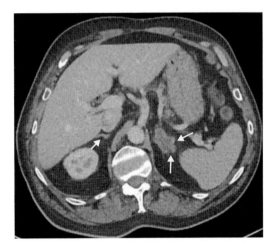

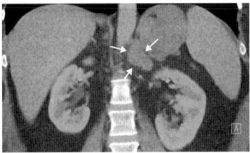

Figure 6.59 Adrenal carcinoma (arrows) in a patient presenting with Cushing's disease.

Figure 6.57 CT scan showing a left adrenal metastasis (arrows). Note normal right adrenal abutting the liver (arrow).

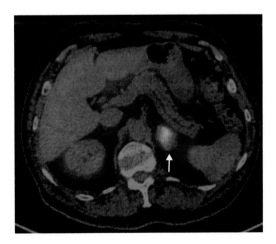

Figure 6.58 PET scan showing active FDG uptake in the left adrenal (arrow).

Adrenal tumours

Adrenal tumours are common. The majority of adrenal tumours are benign and are discovered incidentally in abdominal imaging for other conditions.

- Adrenal adenomas
- Phaeochromocytoma
- Adrenal metastases
- Adrenal carcinoma

Adrenal adenomas are the most common adrenal lesion. They are often an incidental finding in abdominal CT examinations. Most adrenal masses are benign but need to be distinguished from adrenal metastases and other adrenal malignancies, especially if there is a history of current or previous malignancy.

Most adrenal adenomas are non-functioning and asymptomatic. Adrenal adenomas that increase hormone production are called functioning adenomas and present with manifestations of excess hormone secretion:

- Excess aldosterone causes Conn's syndrome. Features include high blood pressure and low potassium levels.
- Excess cortisol causes Cushing's syndrome. Features include high blood pressure, diabetes, and obesity.
- Excess androgens cause virilization. Features include hair growth, increased muscle mass, acne, and abnormal menstrual periods in women.
- Excess oestrogens cause feminization. Features include breast growth and impotence in men.

Radiological features

- CT: 70% of adrenal adenoma are lipid-rich; these are low density on unenhanced CT. 30% of adrenal adenoma are lipid-poor; these are differentiated from non-adenoma by their rapid washout of contrast on enhanced CT.
- MRI: can demonstrate adrenal adenomas as signal dropout on opposed-phase sequences due to the sensitivity of chemical shift MRI to the presence of intracellular fat.

Phaeochromocytoma

Pheochromocytomas are rare, neuroendocrine tumours arising from the adrenal medulla. Classically they can precipitate life-threatening hypertension or cardiac arrhythmias because of excessive catecholamine secretion. Phaeochromocytomas are said to follow a 10% rule because they are associated with a 10% risk of malignancy, 10% are bilateral, 10% are hormonally inactive and 10% are extra-adrenal. Tumours are usually larger than 3 cm at presentation. They are highly vascular and prone to haemorrhage and necrosis. They are characteristically high signal intensity on T2-weighted MRI.

Adrenal metastases

Adrenal metastases are the most common malignant lesions involving the adrenal glands. They are often present at autopsy of patients with known malignant tumours. Adrenal metastases have no specific imaging feature.

Adrenal carcinoma

Adrenal carcinomas are rare and may be functional hormone secreting tumours. They have an irregular shape with mixed density on scanning. Small tumours may be suitable for reaction.

7

Musculoskeletal system

Skeletal system: procedures

Plain films

Plain films still remain the initial radiological investigation of the skeletal system. Views should always be obtained in two projections to avoid missing pathology, such as fractures, oriented in the plane of acquisition.

Isotopes

Technetium-99m phosphonate compounds accumulate in bone several hours after intravenous injection of the isotope; they are principally used for:

- detection of osteomyelitis and other musculoskeletal soft tissue inflammatory changes which involve increased bone turnover;
- metastatic bone lesions: changes are seen much earlier than plain films;
- staging tumours such as breast carcinoma or bronchial carcinoma;
- functional bone abnormality: Paget's disease.

Uptake of the isotope does occur, however, in many other conditions, including osteoarthritis and inflammatory arthropathies.

Arthrography

- Iodine (CT and fluoroscopy) and gadolinium (MRI) based contrast agents are injected into joints such as the knee, hip, elbow, shoulder, wrist and temporomandibular joints to diagnose loose bodies, ligamentous and cartilaginous abnormalities.
- The technique may be followed by computed tomography (CT) or MRI scanning to further evaluate the joint.

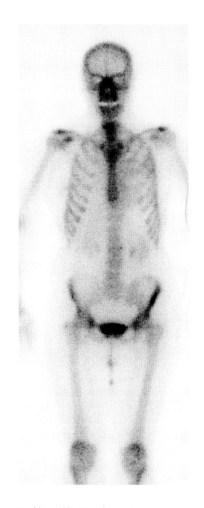

Figure 7.1 Normal isotope bone scan.

- The advent of higher resolution 1.5 T and 3 T MRI has enabled good visualization of hip and shoulder labrum and wrist ligaments without contrast and is now the preferred initial modality in the majority of cases.

Radiology: Lecture Notes, Fourth Edition. Pradip R. Patel.
© 2020 John Wiley & Sons Ltd. Published 2020 by John Wiley & Sons Ltd.
Companion website: www.wiley.com/go/patel/radiology

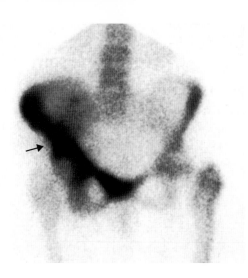

Figure 7.2 Paget's disease: increased isotope uptake in the right pelvis (arrow).

Ultrasound

Ultrasound is utilized for the evaluation of:

- neonatal hip for congenital dislocation;
- soft tissue lesions, abscesses and masses;
- joint effusions;
- joints, tendons, ligaments. The dynamic nature of ultrasound allows for the assessment of joint impingement syndromes around the shoulder (superior and internal) and hips (iliotibial band snapping and iliopsoas tendon snapping) in particular.

Ultrasound-guided intervention

The high special resolution, non-invasive (no radiation dose) and real-time imaging of ultrasound provide for an ideal imaging modality to assist image-guided intervention.

Aspiration of fluid collections such as seromas and abscesses.

Diagnostic and therapeutic injections of bursae mainly around the shoulders, hips and knees.

Injection of sub-centimetre lesions such as Morton's neuroma.

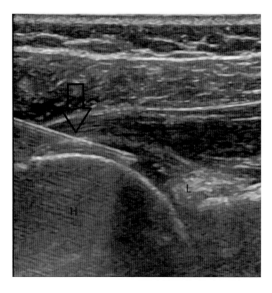

Figure 7.4 Ultrasound-guided injection of the posterior glenohumeral joint. Note the needle (arrow) entering the joint space, posterior labrum (L) and the humeral head (H).

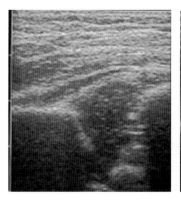
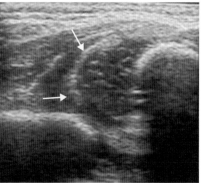

Figure 7.3 Ultrasound of hip in the neonate: normal and dislocated hip (arrows).

Computed tomography (CT)

CT aids:

- assessment of bone tumours prior to surgery, although MRI is now the preferred technique; CT allows for characterization of the matrix mineralization of lesions and clearer definition of cortical involvement. CT is particularly helpful in delineating osteoid osteomas and atypical haemangiomas of the spine.
- evaluation of certain fractures, such as the acetabulum and calcaneum; reconstructions in different planes assist the orthopaedic surgeon to assess a fracture and the need for internal fixation; Modern image manipulation allows for multiplanar review and 3D reconstruction of images.

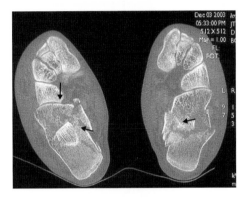

Figure 7.5 CT: bilateral calcaneal fractures involving the articular surfaces (arrows).

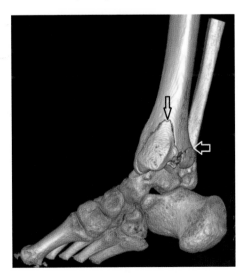

Figure 7.6 Dimensional CT rendered imaging: medial malleolus (vertical arrow) and posterior malleolar (horizontal arrow) fractures.

CT-guided injection to deep joints such as the facet joints or sacroiliac joints.

Magnetic resonance imaging (MRI)

MRI assists the investigation of bone tumours, soft tissue masses, the spinal column and joints. MRI is extremely sensitive in injuries to cartilage, muscle, ligaments and tendons, and has now assumed a central role in the diagnosis of these structures.

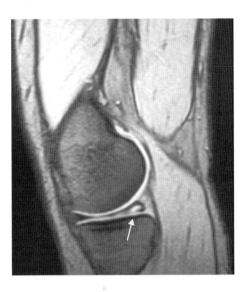

Figure 7.7 MRI knee: meniscal tear affecting the inferior surface of the posterior horn of the meniscus (arrow).

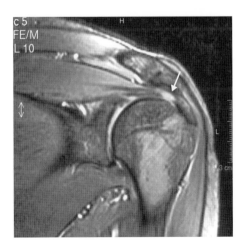

Figure 7.8 MRI shoulder: complete tear of the supraspinatus tendon (arrow).

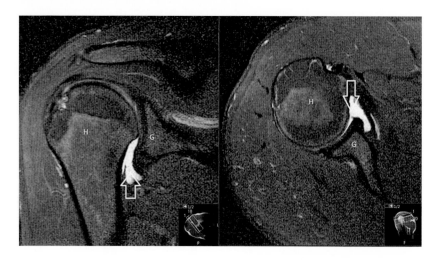

Figure 7.9 MRI shoulder arthrogram: saline (white arrow) outlines the adjacent glenoid labrum attached to the glenoid (G). Humeral head (H).

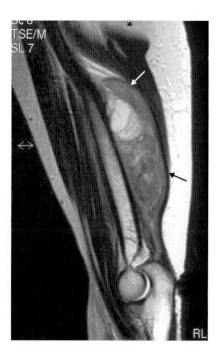

Figure 7.10 MRI arm: sarcoma affecting the triceps muscle (arrows).

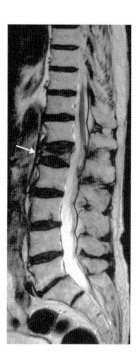

Figure 7.11 MRI lumbar spine showing vertebral collapse (arrow).

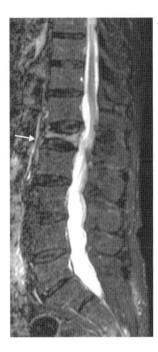

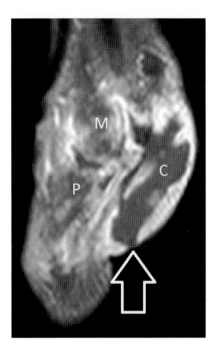

Figure 7.12 The value of MRI in demonstrating that the collapse is recent due to the fact that there is increased signal on this sequence from marrow oedema (arrow).

Figure 7.13 Septic arthritis of the great toe. Sagittal, contrast-enhanced imaging demonstrates a well-defined collection (C) underlying a skin ulcer (arrow). Metacarpal (M) and proximal phalanx (P).

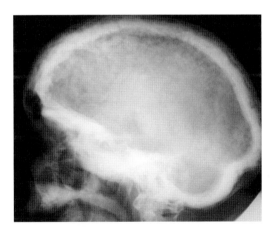

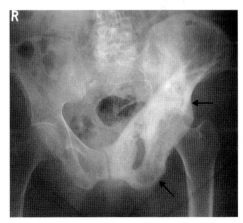

Figure 7.14 Paget's disease: calvarial thickening producing a 'cotton wool' appearance.

Figure 7.15 Paget's disease of the left pelvis with marked, contiguous bone expansion (arrows).

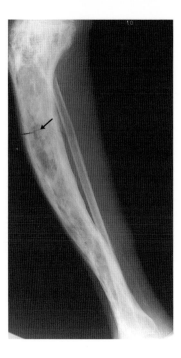

Figure 7.16 Bowing of the tibia with pseudofracture (arrow) in Paget's disease.

Paget's disease

A common disorder of bone architecture, of unknown aetiology, which occurs with increasing frequency after middle age. It is characterized initially by bone resorption, followed by a reparative process in which increased bone deposition results in bone expansion and abnormal modelling.

Presentation

Majority are asymptomatic and diagnosed as an incidental finding: bone pain; fractures; deformity of long bones and skull.

Radiological features

Any bone may be affected.

- Skull. Initially a large area of well-defined bone loss may be seen (osteoporosis circumscripta); later, generalized sclerosis with diploic thickening produces a characteristic 'cotton wool' appearance. There may be an increase in the size of the head.
- Spine. Most commonly involves a single vertebra with sclerosis, altered trabecular pattern and enlargement of the vertebral body.

- Pelvis. Frequently affected with coarsened trabecular pattern, cortical thickening and enlargement of the pubis and ischium.
- Long bones. Widening of bone with deformities, bowing of the tibia and incomplete fractures because of bone softening.

Complications

- Pathological fractures: tend to be sharply transverse.
- Pseudofractures: incomplete fractures found on the convex surfaces of bowed bones.
- Secondary degenerative changes: the hip joint is most frequently involved.
- Malignant degeneration: in widespread Paget's disease, there is an increased incidence of malignant bone tumours, especially osteogenic sarcoma.
- Neurological: nerve entrapment by bone expansion: deafness from VIIIth nerve involvement, encroachment of the spinal exit foramina, etc.
- Cardiovascular: increased shunting of blood in involved bone may cause high output failure, although this is rare.

Key point

In a patient with known Paget's disease, increasing bone pain must raise the suspicion of a fracture, or more importantly development of an osteosarcoma

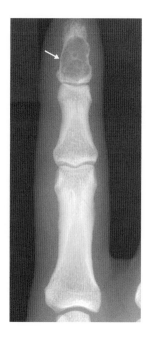

Figure 7.17 Chondroma: a benign cartilaginous tumour (arrow). Note the speckled condroid matrix.

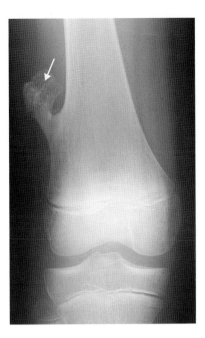

Figure 7.18 Osteochondroma (arrow).

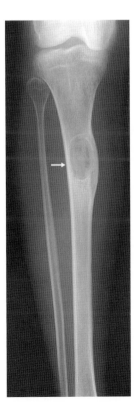

Figure 7.19 Chondromyxoid fibroma (arrow), a rare tumour but demonstrates the features of a benign tumour.

Benign bone tumour

Benign bone tumours are generally well defined and have a narrow zone of transition between normal and abnormal bone. They cause signs and symptoms by expansion and pressure on adjacent structures. If cystic, a pathological fracture may ensue.

Cartilage tumours
Chondroma

A cartilaginous tumour, one of the most common benign tumours of bone, appears as a well-defined lytic lesion, often expanded, with small flecks of calcification. The hands and feet are most frequently affected. Chondromas are often single but may be multiple in Ollier's disease.

Osteochondroma

Probably the commonest benign tumour, containing both bone and cartilage, often on a bony stalk with a bulbous broad distal end. The tumour is often found growing away from a joint, the most frequent site being the metaphyseal region of the lower femur and upper tibia. Hereditary multiple osteochondromas occur in diaphyseal aclasia, where a risk of malignant transformation to chondrosarcoma exists. MRI is particularly helpful in evaluation of tumour transformation or complication (soft tissue impingement and adventitial bursa formation) associated with such lesions.

Bone-forming tumours
Osteoma

A benign tumour that contains only compact osseous tissue, most commonly found in the skull and sinuses. They are round, well defined and appear as a mass of amorphous dense bone with no cartilaginous component.

Osteoid osteoma

A small circular lucent area (nidus) under the cortex surrounded by thickened reactive bone and associated with periosteal reaction. Osteoid osteoma, usually a tumour less than 15 mm in diameter, is generally a lesion of young adults and presents with local pain.

Other benign lesions
Giant cell tumour

A benign tumour, with approximately half discovered in the vicinity of the knee joint. This is a lytic lesion of the epiphyseal region, with cortical thickening, expansion and the potential of turning into a malignant neoplasm.

Osteoblastoma; bone cyst; non-ossifying fibroma; aneurysmal bone cyst; chondromyxoid fibroma

> **Key point**
>
> Pain in the region of a benign lesion such as an osteochondroma should lead to a suspicion of malignant change

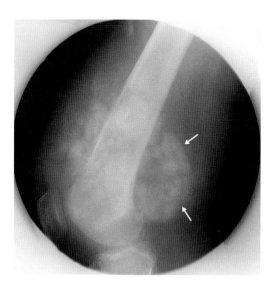

Figure 7.20 Osteogenic sarcoma extending into the soft tissues (arrows).

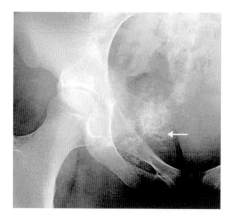

Figure 7.21 Chondrosarcoma of the right pubic ramus (arrow).

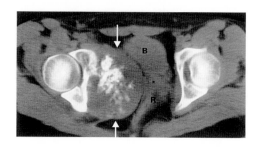

Figure 7.22 CT scan demonstrating the tumour (arrows). B, bladder; R, rectum.

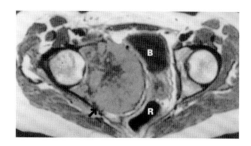

Figure 7.23 MRI showing a large soft tissue component (arrow). B, bladder; R, rectum.

Malignant bone tumour

Primary malignant bone tumours are uncommon: they are destructive, often associated with periosteal reactions, and have a wide zone of transition between normal and abnormal bone. The most common malignant bone tumour is a metastasis and it is often solitary.

Radiological features

Plain films may show an area of bone destruction.

CT and MRI are the best imaging modalities to evaluate tumours and determine bone and soft tissue involvement; definitive diagnosis is by a biopsy. Features that may be verified by CT/MRI are: tumour vascularity; infiltration of surrounding tissues; relationship to nerves and vessels.

Malignant bone tumours

Osteosarcoma

- The second most common primary malignant tumour of bone after multiple myeloma.
- Osteosarcoma presents between the ages of 10 and 25.

- Approximately half appear around the knee joint, involving the metaphysis of the distal femur and proximal tibia.
- It erodes from its origins in the medulla through the cortex, with a resulting soft tissue mass.
- Metastases often spread to the lungs and may form bone.

The classical findings of osteosarcoma are:

- irregular medullary destruction;
- periosteal reaction;
- cortical destruction;
- soft tissue mass;
- new bone formation.

Chondrosarcoma

A slow-growing malignant tumour, derived from cartilage cells, which may contain areas of calcification within the tumour.

- Central type: usually arise from a tubular bone, is lytic and situated in the region of the metaphysis.
- Peripheral type: probably originate from the periosteum or evolve from a previous benign osteochondroma.

Ewing's tumour

- Presents between the ages of 5 and 15 years.
- A highly malignant tumour originating from bone marrow and associated with layered periosteal reactions (onion skin).
- The appearances may mimic an osteomyelitis.

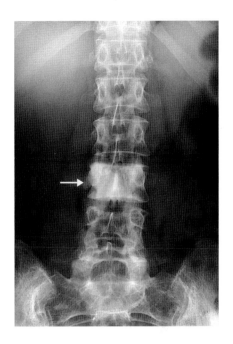

Figure 7.25 Sclerotic deposit in a vertebral body (arrow).

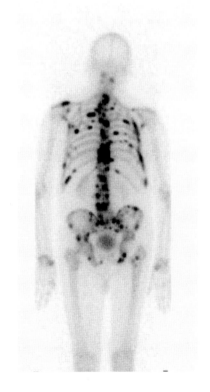

Figure 7.26 Isotope bone scan showing multiple bone deposits.

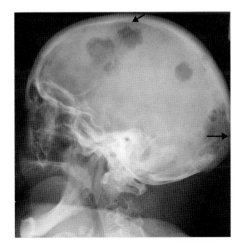

Figure 7.24 Lytic deposits in the cranial vault (arrows).

Bone metastases

Bone metastases are the most common malignant bone tumours. Metastases disseminate mainly to marrow-containing bones; therefore, they are more commonly found in the axial skeleton. Generally, spread distal to the knee and elbow is less likely than the proximal skeleton. Any primary tumour may metastasize to bone, but the most frequent to do so are the following.

- Breast: high incidence of bone deposits, usually lytic in nature but may be sclerotic or mixed; the commonest cause of sclerotic deposits in females.
- Prostate: almost always sclerotic, lytic deposits being rare; the commonest cause of sclerotic deposits in a male.
- Lung: lytic deposits; peripheral deposits in the hands and feet are rare, but if present are likely to be from a bronchial carcinoma.
- Kidney, thyroid: lytic and can be highly vascular with bone expansion.
- Adrenal gland: predominantly lytic.

Presentation

Bone pain; pathological fracture; soft tissue swelling; staging or during follow-up of primary tumours.

Radiological features

Bone metastases tend to be either lytic or sclerotic. The following can be seen on plain films.

- Lytic deposits. Destruction of bone detail with poor definition of margins and associated pathological fractures are the principal features. Periosteal reactions are rare compared to primary malignant tumours.
- Sclerotic deposits. Show as an area of ill-defined increased density with subsequent loss of bone architecture. Vertebral secondaries may feature sclerotic pedicles. With multiple lesions, a diagnosis of metastases is almost certain. Isotope bone scanning is more sensitive than plain films (localized areas of increased uptake: hot spots).

In cases where the primary tumour is unknown, an image-guided biopsy of the bone lesion may reveal the site of the primary carcinoma.

Differential diagnosis

- Paget's disease (sclerotic areas).
- Multiple myeloma (lytic areas).
- Primary malignant tumour.
- Infection or osteomyelitis.

> **Key point**
>
> Radionuclide imaging is much more sensitive detecting metastases than plain film imaging

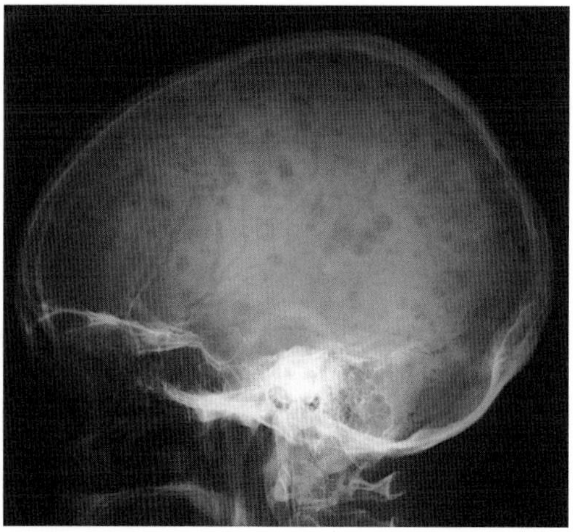

Figure 7.27 Lateral skull in multiple myeloma showing widespread well-defined 'punched out' lytic lesions in the cranial vault.

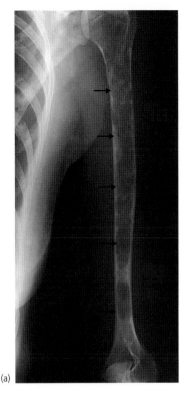
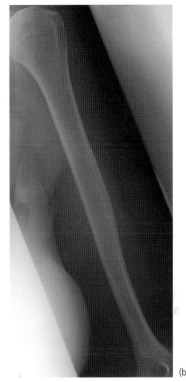

(a)   (b)

Figure 7.28 Myeloma deposits (arrows) in the humerus (a) producing lytic areas and 'endosteal scalloping'; compare the appearances with a normal humerus (b).

Multiple myeloma

Multiple myeloma is a primary malignant tumour of bone marrow in which there is infiltration of the marrow-producing areas of the skeleton by a malignant proliferation of plasma cells. The skull, spine, pelvis, ribs, scapulae and the proximal axial skeleton are primarily involved with destruction of marrow and erosion of bony trabeculae; the distal skeleton is rarely involved. The disease may occur in a disseminated form or as a localized solitary enlarging mass (plasmacytoma). Multiple myeloma is the most common primary malignant tumour of bone and tends to be confined to the skeletal system.

Presentation

A male predominance, usually in the over-40 age group; weight loss; malaise; bone pain; backache; vertebral body collapse; pathological fracture; Bence–Jones proteinuria.

Radiological features

At the time of presentation, 80–90% have skeletal abnormalities. Plain films feature the following.

- Generalized osteoporosis with a prominence of the bony trabecular pattern, especially in the spine, resulting from marrow involvement with myeloma tissue. Loss of spinal bone density may be the only radiological sign in multiple myeloma. Pathological fractures are common.
- Compression fractures of the vertebral bodies, indistinguishable from those of senile osteoporosis.
- Scattered, 'punched-out' lytic lesions with well-defined margins, those lying near the cortex produce internal scalloping.
- Bone expansion with extension through the cortex, producing soft tissue masses.

Complications

- Pathological fractures that heal with abundant callus.
- Hypercalcaemia secondary to excessive bone destruction.

- Renal failure may result from a combination of amyloid deposition, hypercalcaemia and tubular precipitation of abnormal proteins.
- Increased incidence of infections such as pneumonia.
- Hyperuricaemia and secondary gout.

> **Key point**
>
> Osteoporosis or vertebral collapse may be the only skeletal manifestation of multiple myeloma

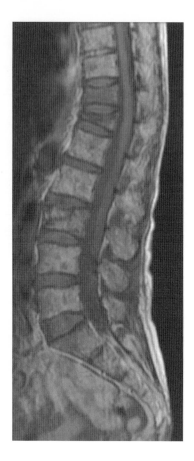

Figure 7.30 Lower thoracic and lumbar vertebrae collapse due to metastatic disease.

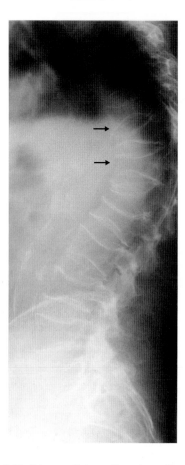

Figure 7.29 Osteoporotic lower thoracic and lumbar spine showing loss of bone density and vertebral collapse (arrows).

Osteoporosis

Osteoporosis is a condition in which there is a reduction of bone mass.

Presentation

- Asymptomatic.
- Bone pain.
- Skeletal fractures.
- Vertebral compression fractures.

Radiological investigations

- Plain films.
- Bone densitometry either by CT (QCT) or dual-energy X-ray absorptiometry (DEXA).

Radiological features

Detection of osteoporosis on plain films requires a reduction in bone mass of at least 30%. Osteoporosis results in a loss of bone density, a decrease in the number of trabeculae and coarse striations.

The condition manifests itself most prominently in the spine. The vertebral bodies appear lucent with thin cortical lines, often with a biconcave appearance ('cod fish' vertebrae), vertebral wedging and collapse; this subsequently leads to a kyphosis. Fractures of the peripheral skeleton, including femoral neck fractures, commonly occur even after minor trauma.

Causes of local osteoporosis

- Disuse of a particular part (tumours, fracture).
- Inflammatory conditions such as rheumatoid arthritis and osteomyelitis.
- Sudeck's atrophy (neural or muscle paralysis). Development of pain and osteoporosis often after slight trauma; it may have a neurovascular aetiology.

Causes of generalized osteoporosis

- Senile osteoporosis.
- Postmenopause.
- Steroid therapy.
- Immobility (prolonged bed rest).
- Endocrine: Cushing's disease, hyperthyroidism.
- Multiple myeloma.
- Nutritional deficiency syndromes: scurvy, malnutrition, chronic liver disease, malabsorption syndromes.

> **Key point**
>
> At least 30–40% bone loss is needed before plain films can detect osteoporosis. Osteoporotic vertebral collapse must be distinguished from metastatic collapse

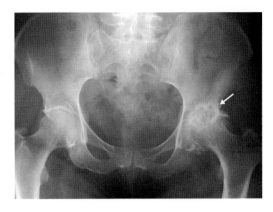

Figure 7.31 Degenerative changes in the left hip with loss of joint space and osteophyte formation (arrow).

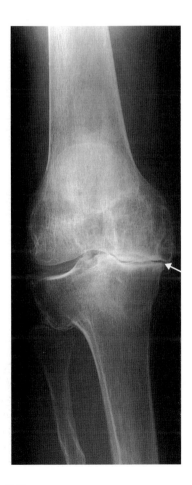

Figure 7.32 Degenerative changes at the knee joint with loss of medial compartment joint space (arrow).

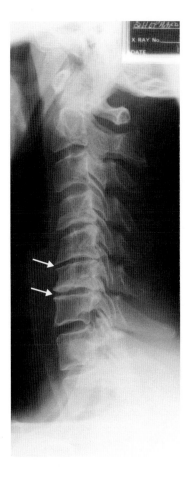

Figure 7.33 Degenerative changes in the cervical spine with mid and lower cervical loss of disc space (arrows).

Osteoarthritis

Osteoarthritis is characterized by degeneration of articular cartilage and is part of the normal ageing process due to wear and tear of the articular surface. Secondary osteoarthritis results from previous trauma with malalignment of articular surfaces, joint infection and rheumatoid arthritis.

Radiological features

Any joint, particularly weight-bearing, may be affected. The hips, knees, shoulders, hands, wrists and spine are frequently involved. Features of osteoarthritis include the following.

- Osteophyte formation: osteophytes are spurs of compact bone that form at joint margins.
- Joint space narrowing: cartilage loss eventually leads to non-uniform joint space narrowing.
- Loose bodies: result from separation of cartilage and osteophytes.
- Subchondral cysts and sclerosis: increased bone density around joints with degenerative cyst formation.

Common sites of involvement

Knee

The most common joint involved, with femorotibial compartment loss of joint space. The medial compartment is the weight-bearing part under greatest stress, and so almost always shows the earliest narrowing. Severe changes may require total knee joint replacement.

Spine

Degenerative changes are present in nearly all elderly patients. Features include:

- narrowing of disc space;
- new bone formation (spurring) between adjacent vertebrae may cause nerve root impingement or spinal cord compression;
- sclerosis and osteophytes at intervertebral apophyseal joints.

Hips

Joint space narrowing is seen initially at the superior maximum weight-bearing aspect, with femoral and acetabular osteophytes. Other findings may include sclerosis and subchondral cyst formation. Severe changes often necessitate total hip joint replacement.

Hands

Typically affects:

- base of first metacarpal;
- proximal interphalangeal (PIP) joints (Bouchard's nodes);
- distal interphalangeal joints (Heberden's nodes).

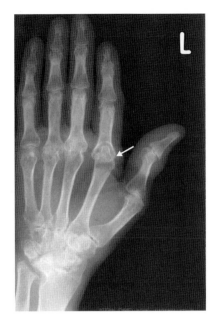 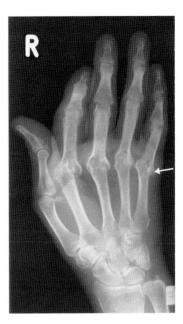

Figure 7.34 Rheumatoid arthritis: erosive changes, predominantly at the metacarpophalangeal joints (arrows) and wrists.

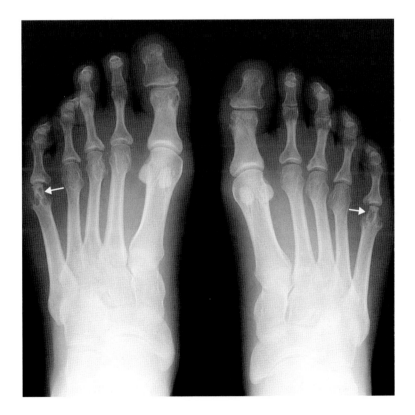

Figure 7.35 Rheumatoid arthritis: symmetrical erosive changes at the heads of the fifth metatarsals (arrows).

Rheumatoid arthritis

Rheumatoid arthritis is defined as a chronic polyarthritis due to inflammation, congestion and proliferation of synovium, leading to bone erosion with cartilage destruction.

Radiological features

Radiological changes lag behind clinical symptoms. Rheumatoid arthritis tends to have a symmetrical distribution, most commonly affecting the hands and feet. Any synovial joint may be involved, the most significant and frequent findings in rheumatoid arthritis being uniform narrowing of joint space, marginal erosions and periarticular osteoporosis.

The following features may be found.

- Joint swelling: from synovial membrane proliferation and joint effusions.
- Erosions: initially located in the periarticular area along the joint margins, where no protective layer exists. Erosions eventually spread across the articular surface.
- Osteoporosis: periarticular at first, but later generalized from disuse and hyperaemia.
- Joint space narrowing: widening of joint spaces at the outset of disease, but eventually a significant narrowing from erosions and cartilage deformity. Obliteration and complete destruction of joint space eventually leads to ankylosis.

Specific sites of involvement

- Hands: the metacarpophalangeal (MCP) and PIP joints are commonly affected, with distal interphalangeal joint involvement less marked. Abnormalities include soft tissue swelling and subluxation at the MCP joints:
  - 'Boutonnière' deformity: flexion deformity at PIP joint and extension at distal interphalangeal joint;
  - 'Swan neck' deformity: hyperextension at PIP joint and flexion at distal interphalangeal joint.
- Feet: broadly similar changes to hands.
- Wrists: erosions with fusion of the carpal bones.
- Elbows: common site for soft tissue rheumatoid nodules.
- Shoulders: erosion of humeral head and acromioclavicular joints.
- Knees: uniform joint-space narrowing with osteoporosis. Baker's cyst is a complication, with rupture producing symptoms and signs similar to those of a deep vein thrombosis.
- Cervical spine: subluxation, erosion and fusion. Subluxation is most common at the atlanto-axial joint.

> **Key point**
>
> The arthropathy of rheumatoid arthritis is generally a symmetrical one

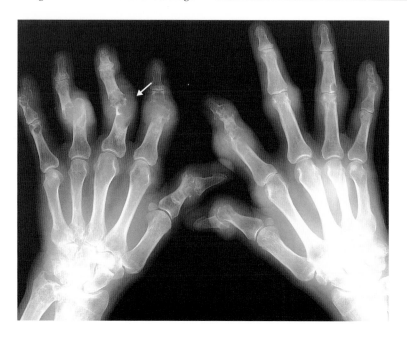

Figure 7.36 Gout: soft tissue swelling with sharply defined erosions (arrow). Involvement is asymmetrical.

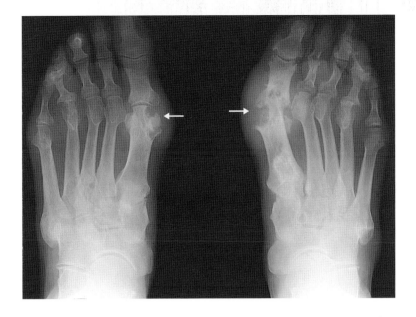

Figure 7.37 Gout affecting the first metatarsophalangeal joints. Soft tissue swelling is present with large erosions (arrows).

Gout

Gout is characterized by a raised plasma uric acid level with recurrent attacks of arthritis. It is due to an inborn error of metabolism and predominantly affects males.

Presentation

- Hot swollen joint, usually the first metatarsophalangeal (MTP) joint.
- Asymptomatic hyperuricaemia.
- Can present like a septic joint with systemic symptoms.

Radiological features

Radiological changes only occur many years after clinical symptoms. There exists a predilection for the first MTP joint, but ankles, knees, elbows and other joints may also be involved. Plain films may reveal the following.

- Joint effusions and swellings.
- Erosions: these tend to have a 'punched-out' appearance, lying separately from the articular surface. Bone density is preserved.
- Tophi: composed of sodium urate and deposited in bone, soft tissues and around joints. Calcification in the tophi may be found, and intraosseous tophi may enlarge to produce erosions with joint destruction.

Complications

Renal calculi: non-opaque on plain films; renal failure.

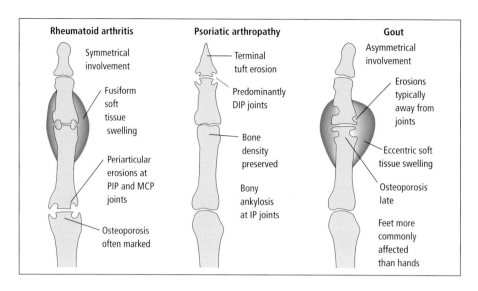

Rheumatoid arthritis	Psoriatic arthropathy	Gout
Symmetrical involvement	Terminal tuft erosion	Asymmetrical involvement
Fusiform soft tissue swelling	Predominantly DIP joints	Erosions typically away from joints
Periarticular erosions at PIP and MCP joints	Bone density preserved	Eccentric soft tissue swelling
Osteoporosis often marked	Bony ankylosis at IP joints	Osteoporosis late
		Feet more commonly affected than hands

Figure 7.38 Differential diagnosis of erosive arthropathy.

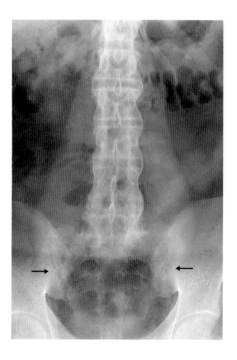

Figure 7.39 Typical 'bamboo spine' with paraspinal ligament calcification. The right sacroiliac joint appears ill defined (→) and the left fused (←).

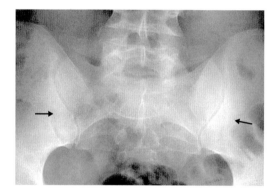

Figure 7.40 Normal sacroiliac joints (arrows).

Ankylosing spondylitis

Ankylosing spondylitis, a progressive inflammatory disease, usually affects young adult males, often with a family history of the disease; 95% of patients carry the human leukocyte antigen (HLA-B27 antigen).

Presentation

- Repeated attacks of backache and stiffness.
- Anorexia and weight loss.

Radiological features

On plain films, the following features may be seen.

- *Sacroiliac joints.* The earliest changes begin in the sacroiliac joints with symmetrical blurring and poor definition of joint margins. Later, erosion and bony sclerosis lead to a tendency for complete sacroiliac joint fusion. Both joints are commonly affected; a unilateral sacroiliitis should raise the suspicion of a bacterial infection, commonly tuberculous. Sacroiliitis is usually evident on bone scanning before any radiographic change.
- *Spinal changes.* The entire spine may be involved but changes usually commence in the lumbar region and progress upwards to involve the thoracic and cervical spine. The features most commonly noted are: squaring of the vertebral bodies due to new bone formation in the anterior vertebral bodies, and filling in of the normal anterior concavity by longitudinal ligamentous calcification; calcification of the lateral and anterior spinal ligaments to produce the classical 'bamboo spine'.
- *Peripheral joint involvement.* An erosive arthropathy may accompany ankylosing spondylitis, the hips being the commonest joints involved.

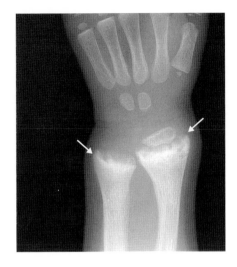

Figure 7.41 Rickets in a 2-year-old child with widening and cupping of the distal radius and ulna (arrows).

Complications/associations

- Upper lobe lung fibrosis.
- Aortic incompetence: from an aortitis of the ascending aorta.
- Ventilatory failure: due to restrictive chest movements and ankylosis of the costovertebral joints.
- Atlanto-axial subluxation.
- Fractures: spinal rigidity causes increased susceptibility to trauma.
- Inflammatory bowel disease: a colitis resembling Crohn's disease or ulcerative colitis.
- Iritis.

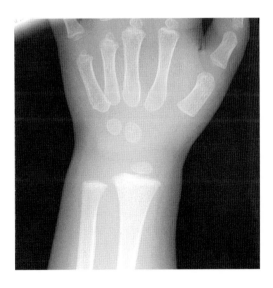

Figure 7.42 Normal appearances in a child of similar age.

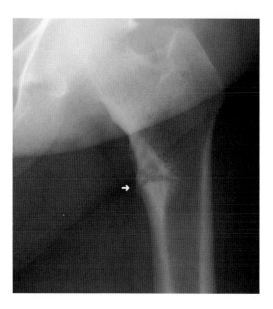

Figure 7.43 'Looser's zone' in the femur (arrow).

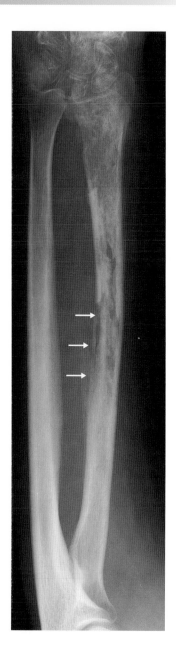

Figure 7.44 Acute osteomyelitis of the radius with patchy bone destruction (arrows).

Rickets

Vitamin D deficiency in children can cause rickets. Deficiency may be nutritional, due to malabsorption, chronic renal disease or prolonged anticonvulsant therapy.

Presentation

Failure to thrive; bone pain; bone deformities.

Radiological features

The principal pathological change is a lack of calcification of osteoid tissue in the growing epiphysis. The whole skeleton is affected, especially rapidly growing areas: wrists, knees and proximal humeri. Greenstick fractures are common.

The following features may be seen on plain films.

- Widening of the growth plate and epiphysis, with delayed appearance of epiphyses.
- Fraying and indistinct margins of the metaphysis producing a cupped appearance.
- Periosteal reactions, especially during the healing stage.
- Bowing and curvature of bones.
- Bulbous enlargement of the anterior ends of the ribs producing a 'rickety rosary'.

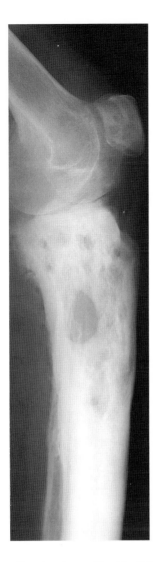

Figure 7.45 Chronic osteomyelitis of the tibia with extensive sclerosis.

Osteomalacia

Vitamin D deficiency in the mature skeleton can lead to osteomalacia, the adult counterpart of rickets.

Presentation

Bone pain; muscular weakness; elevated serum alkaline phosphatase; pathological fractures.

Radiological features

- Generalized reduction in bone density.
- Looser's zones (pseudofractures) are narrow translucent bands, at the cortical margins, and are diagnostic of osteomalacia. They are seen most frequently in the ribs, scapulae, pubic rami and medial aspects of the proximal femora.
- Biconcave vertebrae ('cod fish' vertebrae).
- Bone softening leading to triradiate pelvis.

Osteomyelitis

Osteomyelitis is an infection of bone, *Staphylococcus aureus* being responsible for the majority of cases; other causes include tuberculosis and *Salmonella* infection in sickle cell disease. The inflammatory process can be either acute or chronic; the latter leading to bone necrosis and pus formation, which sometimes discharges through to the skin to form a sinus communication with bone. Necrotic bone may separate from living tissue to produce a sequestrum. Sources of infection may be:

- haematogenous: usually in children;
- direct traumatic implantation, e.g. compound fracture or surgery;
- extension from adjacent soft tissues, e.g. a foot ulcer in diabetes.

Presentation

- Pain.
- Pyrexia.

Radiological features

- *Plain films*: may be normal for up to 10 days but the earliest sign is soft tissue swelling. Infected bone initially loses detail and becomes ill-defined with periosteal reaction and eventually bone destruction.
- *Isotope bone scanning*: uses technetium, gallium or labelled white cells. All indicate increased activity but are non-specific, as conditions such as Paget's disease or neoplasia may also show increased uptake. The findings have to be interpreted in the clinical setting.
- *CT*: detects associated soft tissue mass and sequestra, which may require surgical removal.

- *MRI*: a sensitive technique in detecting infection. This will often show joint effusion and marrow oedema/cortical breach underlying a skin ulcer. MRI is particularly helpful in detecting haematogenous septic involvement of the joint in the paediatric population.

Chronic osteomyelitis

Organisms responsible for the infection persist in dead bone, and exacerbations may ensue periodically. The bone appears thickened and sclerotic with a central radiolucent destructive area, often with a chronic draining sinus. An abscess with a sclerotic margin, sometimes containing a sequestrum, may follow (Brodie's abscess).

Complications

- Soft tissue abscess.
- Fistulae.
- Premature fusion of epiphyses.
- Deformity.
- Pyogenic arthritis leading to bony ankylosis (e.g. hip fusion).

Key point

MRI and nuclear medicine scans detect changes of acute osteomyelitis much earlier than plain films

8

Trauma

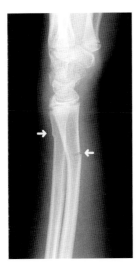

Figure 8.1 Greenstick fractures of the distal forearm (arrows).

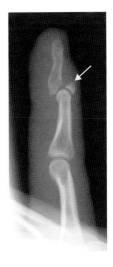

Figure 8.2 Small avulsion fracture at the base of the distal phalanx (arrow).

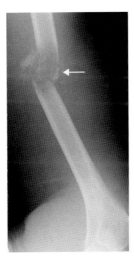

Figure 8.3 Secondary deposit in the humerus; pathological fracture (arrow).

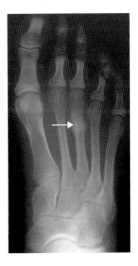

Figure 8.4 Healing stress fracture of the third metatarsal (arrow).

Radiology: Lecture Notes, Fourth Edition. Pradip R. Patel.
© 2020 John Wiley & Sons Ltd. Published 2020 by John Wiley & Sons Ltd.
Companion website: www.wiley.com/go/patel/radiology

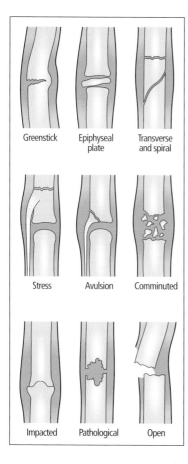

Figure 8.5 Types of fracture.

- Comminuted: a fracture with multiple fragments.
- Avulsion: a fragment of bone becomes detached from the site of a ligamentous or tendon insertion.
- Pathological: a fracture through diseased bone, often after trivial trauma, e.g. Paget's disease, osteoporosis or tumour.
- Stress or fatigue fracture: results from chronic repetitive minor trauma. Susceptible areas include the second and third metatarsals (March fracture), proximal tibial shaft, fibula and the femoral shaft (long-distance runners and ballet dancers).
- Impacted fracture: the fragments are compressed into each other, with no apparent visible fracture line.
- Epiphyseal plate fractures in children under the age of 16. These can be classified into types 1 to 5 using the Salter Harris classification.

Complications of fractures

- Non-union: results from inadequate immobilization or the presence of a pathological fracture.
- Mal-union: healing with poor angulation.
- Avascular necrosis: disruption of the blood supply leads to bone death; the most common sites to be affected are the femoral head, proximal pole of the scaphoid and the head of the talus.
- Osteoarthritis: early degenerative changes in a joint resulting from poor malalignment.
- Osteoporosis: from disuse, and in its most severe form, Sudeck's atrophy, may be associated with pain and soft tissue swelling.

Fractures

Plain films are the principal method of initial evaluation of a patient with suspected skeletal trauma. Any bone may fracture but some are particularly susceptible. Typical signs and features of a fracture are as follows.

- Fracture line: the fracture line may traverse the whole diameter of the bone or minor fractures may cause a break in the continuity of the normal cortical outline.
- Soft tissue swelling: usually accompanies a fracture.
- Cortical irregularity: a slight bulge or step in the cortex.

Types of fracture

- Greenstick: in children, bone tends to be flexible and so a fracture may occur with bending of bone on one side with a break of the cortex on the other side. The bone may also buckle without an actual break (torus fracture).

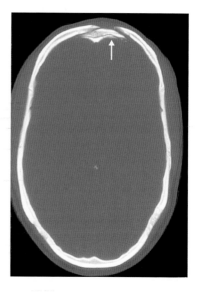

Figure 8.6 CT: depressed skull fracture (arrow).

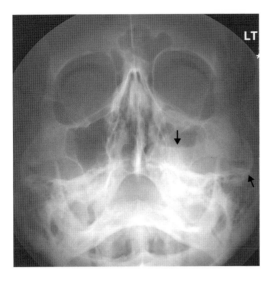

Figure 8.7 Facial bone fracture: fluid level in the maxillary antrum (↓) and zygomatic arch fracture (→).

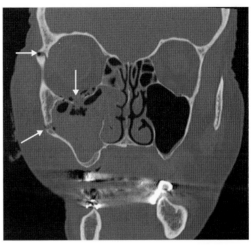

Figure 8.8 CT facial bones showing fractures of the inferior orbital wall, maxillary antrum and origin of the zygomatic arch (tripod fracture; arrows).

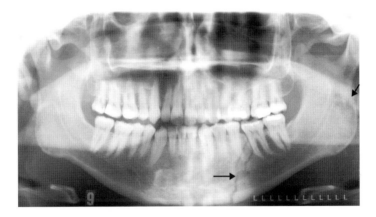

Figure 8.9 Orthopantomogram: fractures of the mandible (arrows).

Facial bone fractures

Skull fractures

The role of plain skull films in the evaluation of trauma has virtually disappeared, as CT scanning is the initial investigation of choice if there is any significant head trauma, especially in the presence of reduced consciousness or any neurological symptoms. CT will detect fractures as well as underlying pathology such as intracerebral haemorrhage or contusions, subdural and extradural collections.

Fractures are seen as follows.

- Linear: sharply defined linear lucencies with the absence of a sclerotic margin.
- Depressed: bony fragment thrust inwards with inner table depressed by greater than the thickness of the cranial vault.

Facial bone fractures

- Occipitomental view taken with the chin tilted upwards.
- Classified into Le Fort 1,11 or 111.

- Zygomatic bone may be fractured from a direct punch to the face. A fluid level in the maxillary antrum associated with the fracture is likely to represent blood. Fracture occurs at several of the four prongs arising from the body:
  - the zygomatic arch;
  - the zygomatico-frontal suture;
  - the inferior wall of the orbit;
  - lateral wall of the maxillary antrum.

Orbital fracture

Orbital floor fracture may result in entrapment of the inferior rectus or herniation of the orbital contents into the maxillary sinus (blowout fracture). This results in restriction of upward gaze.

Mandibular fractures

A blow to the mandible often results in a fracture at two sites as the mandible can be considered as a bony ring. The fracture may involve any part of the mandible – the symphysis, body, angle, ramus or condyle.

Nasal bone fractures

Common and needs an X-ray only if there is deformity.

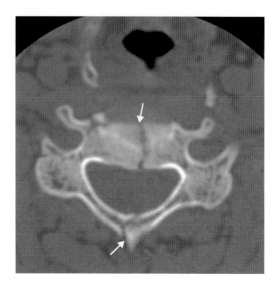

Figure 8.11 CT: fractures of the cervical spine (arrows).

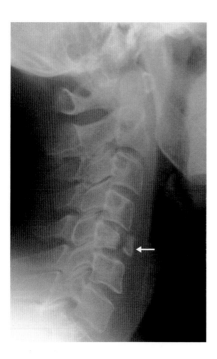

Figure 8.10 Fracture of the C5 vertebral body (arrow).

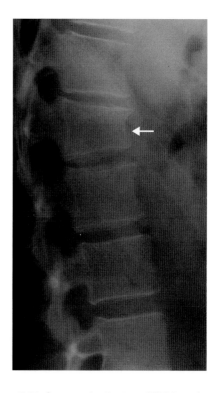

Figure 8.12 Compression fracture of T12 (arrow).

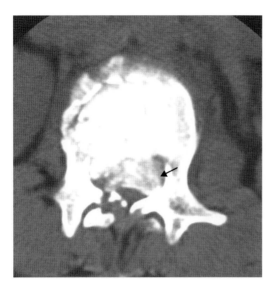

Figure 8.13 Severe vertebral fracture with a bony fragment in the spinal canal (arrow).

Spinal fractures

Cervical spine

- Projections – AP, lateral, open mouth view (to see C1 and C2), oblique views to evaluate the facet joints and intervertebral foramina. Flexion and extension views to diagnose instability, performed with caution.
- Check alignment and all seven cervical vertebrae are visualized, noting any step deformities.

The following fractures and dislocations of the cervical spine may occur.

- *Atlanto-axial subluxation*: the space between the odontoid peg and the posterior part of C1 should be no more than 3 mm in adults and 5 mm in children.
- *Jefferson's fracture*: lateral burst fracture of C1 resulting from a compression injury to the vertex of the skull (diving injury).
- *Odontoid peg fractures*: most commonly through the base of the odontoid peg.
- *Hangman's fracture*: hyperextension injury to C2 causing pedicle fractures.

- *Teardrop fracture*: small fragment avulsed from the lower anterior vertebral body (flexion injury with anterior compression).
- *Vertebral body fracture*: compression fracture of the body.

Vertebral body fracture

Unless there is osteoporotic change, only a severe injury will result in a vertebral body fracture. The thoracolumbar region from T11 to L2, at the level of the conus medullaris, is relatively susceptible to injury. The canal diameter of thoracic spine is narrower than the cervical or lumbar spine, hence a smaller amount of space is available before cord compression occurs.

- *Burst fracture* – bony segment shatters and displaces in all directions.
- *Wedge fracture* – compression with loss of height and anterior wedging.
- *Fracture dislocation* – both fracture and dislocation take place simultaneously.

CT or MRI scanning will accurately detect the presence of the fracture and any impingement on the spinal canal. Bone fragments may be displaced posteriorly into the spinal canal causing neurological symptoms.

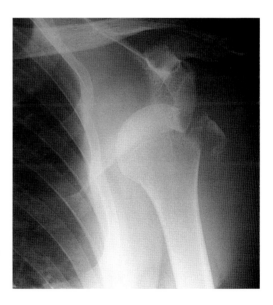

Figure 8.14 Anterior dislocation with a fracture of the greater tuberosity.

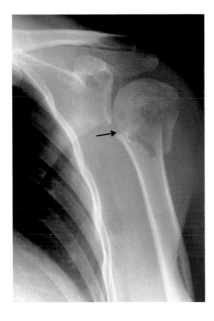

Figure 8.15 Humeral neck fracture (arrow).

Shoulder dislocation

- Dislocation commonly results from an athletic injury or fall.
- Almost always occurs anteriorly with the humeral head lying in front and below the glenoid cavity.
- Posterior dislocation is rare and sometimes difficult to identify.
- Avulsion of the glenoid labrum or avulsion of the greater tuberosity may be associated with the dislocation.
- Recurrent dislocations may give rise to a 'hatchet defect', a concave depression in the humeral head, resulting from humeral head collision with the inferior glenoid.
- Axillary artery and nerve are at risk of damage.

Humeral neck fracture

- Surgical neck fractures are the most common fracture of the proximal humerus.
- Anatomic neck fractures have higher incidence of avascular necrosis.
- Displacement of 1 cm or more between fracture fragments generally needs surgical treatment.

- Undisplaced stable fractures, with active movement and little pain and no abnormal motion between fragments, treated conservatively with the arm in a sling.
- Axillary artery and nerve are at risk of damage.

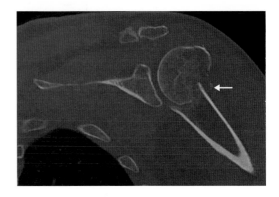

Figure 8.16 CT humeral neck fracture (arrow).

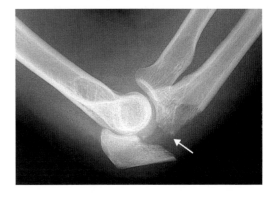

Figure 8.17 Olecranon fracture (arrow).

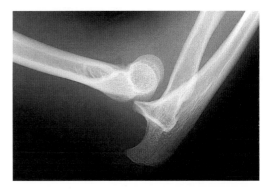

Figure 8.18 Dislocation at the elbow.

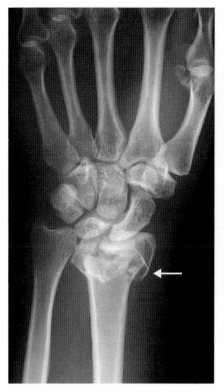 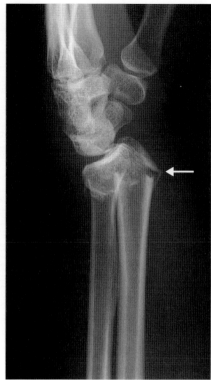

Figure 8.19 Colles' fracture (arrows).

Elbow fractures

These can be classified as follows.

- *Supracondylar fractures*, common in children. Complications include nerve injuries (median and radial). Brachial artery injury should always be suspected with supracondylar fractures. Although rare, the most serious complication is Volkmann ischemic contracture from muscle and nerve necrosis and eventual replacement by fibrotic tissue producing contracture.
- *Intercondylar T and Y fractures*: complex fractures of the codyles which are more difficult to treat.
- *Lateral and medial condylar fracture*.
- *Radial head and neck fracture*: the mechanism is usually a fall onto an outstretched hand. The most common of all fractures of the elbow.

- *Olecranon fracture*, usually from direct blow or a fall onto an outstretched hand. Ulnar nerve injury is common.
- *Elbow dislocation*.

Colles' fracture

- May follow a fall onto the outstretched hand, resulting in a fracture of the lower end of the radius with posterior displacement of the distal fragment.
- Dinner fork deformity with posterior angulation of distal radius.
- Often associated with a fracture of the ulnar styloid process.
- Manual reduction, immobilization or open reduction.
- Smith's fracture – anterior angulation of distal radius.

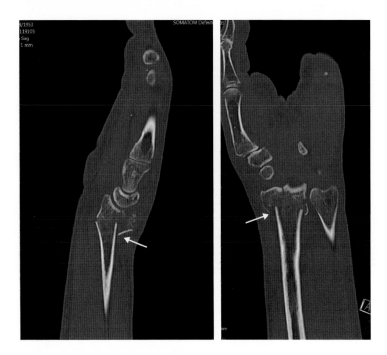

Figure 8.20 Colles' fracture (arrows).

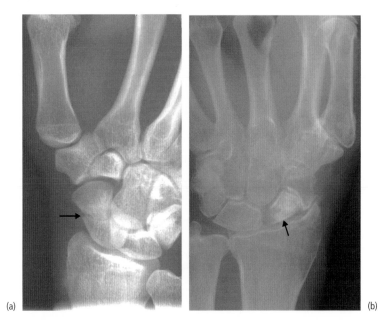

(a)

(b)

Figure 8.21 (a) Scaphoid fracture (arrow); (b) scaphoid fracture resulting in sclerosis of the proximal fragment due to avascular necrosis (arrow).

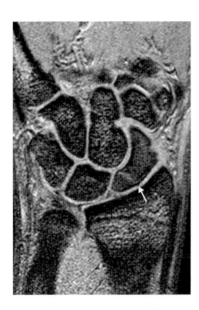

Figure 8.22 MRI scan demonstrating a subtle scaphoid fracture, not demonstrated on plain films.

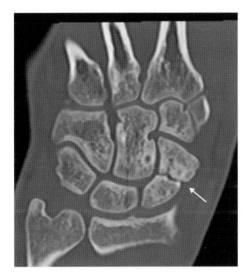

Figure 8.23 CT showing ununited scaphoid fracture.

Scaphoid fracture

This is the most commonly fractured carpal bone. The fracture is often difficult to identify and if there is clinical suspicion, a further X-ray after 10 days is required, when it may be more easily visualized. MRI is useful to identify subtle and occult fractures and to detect early avascular changes.

Treatment

- Non-displaced waist fractures – cast 6–8 weeks.
- Displaced waist fracture – internal screw fixation.
- Proximal pole fractures – internal fixation.
- Distal pole fractures – cast immobilization.

Complications

- Non-union – weakness and pain.
- Secondary degenerative change.

The blood supply to the bone is from distal to proximal and so complications such as non-union and avascular necrosis of the proximal fragment are frequently seen.

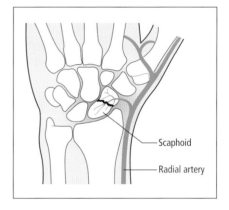

Figure 8.24 Blood supply to scaphoid.

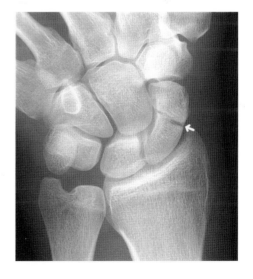

Figure 8.25 Scaphoid fracture (arrow).

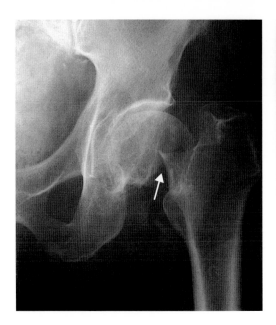

Figure 8.26 Femoral neck fracture (arrow).

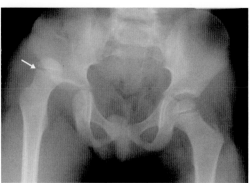

Figure 8.28 Traumatic dislocation of the right hip (arrow).

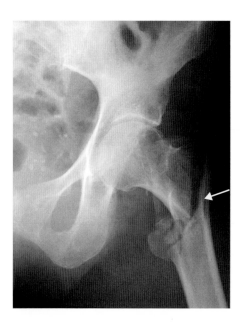

Figure 8.27 Intertrochanteric fracture (arrow).

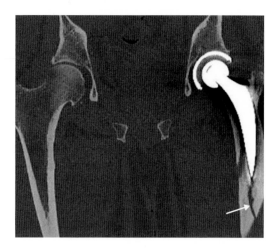

Figure 8.29 Fracture at the site of a hip prosthesis (arrow).

Hip fractures

- Most hip fractures in the elderly (90%) occur as a result of a minor fall and in younger individuals following high-impact trauma.
- Hip fractures are associated with significant morbidity and mortality, with 15–20% of patients dying within one year of fracture.
- Conditions that predispose to hip fractures include ageing, osteoporosis and osteomalacia.
- The vascular supply to the proximal femur is tenuous and femoral neck fractures often disrupt the blood supply to the head of the femur. The medial circumflex artery supplies the majority of the blood supply to the head and neck.

Fractures can be classified into several categories.

Intracapsular

These have a higher incidence of avascular necrosis and non-union (35%).

- *Subcapital*: most common intracapsular fracture, often impacted under the head of the femur, sometimes seen just as a white line of increased density and often leads to avascular necrosis of the head. MRI or isotope bone scan may be useful to confirm subtle fractures.
- *Transcervical*: across the neck of the femur, frequently associated with varus deformity.

Extracapsular

- *Intertrochanteric*: fracture through a line between the greater and lesser trochanters. Intertrochanteric fractures are often associated with a varus deformity.
- *Subtrochanteric*: sited below the lesser trochanter.

Figure 8.30 Blood supply to femoral head.

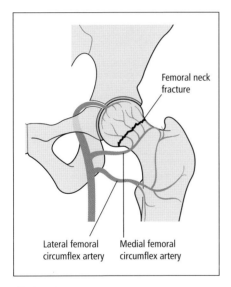

Femoral neck
fracture

Lateral femoral
circumflex artery

Medial femoral
circumflex artery

Figure 8.31 (a) Fracture of the patella (arrow); (b) tibial plateau fracture (arrow).

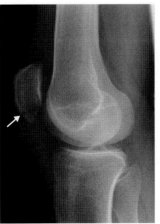

(a)

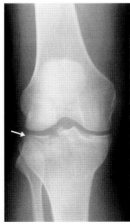

(b)

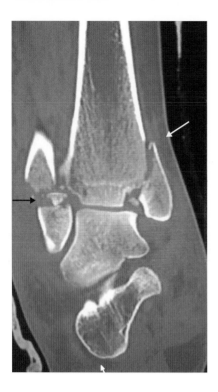

Figure 8.32 CT reconstruction of the ankle fractures (arrows).

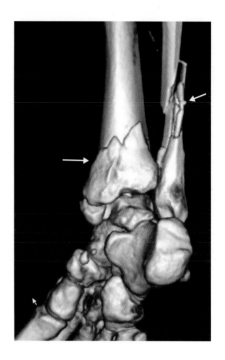

Figure 8.33 CT 3D reconstruction of the fractures (arrows).

Knee fractures

Tibial plateau fracture

- Caused by axial loading with valgus or varus forces, such as in a fall from a height or collision with the bumper of a car.
- Patient is generally unable to bear weight.
- The lateral tibial plateau is most commonly fractured and usually results in a depression of the tibial plateau.
- May need elevation with surgical internal fixation.
- Often associated with damage to the cruciate or collateral ligaments.
- CT or MRI scans may be necessary to fully delineate the extent of tibial plateau fractures, other complex knee fractures and soft tissue injury.

Patella fracture

- Caused by a direct blow, such as a dashboard injury in a motor vehicle accident or a fall on a flexed knee.
- Also caused by forceful quadriceps contraction while the knee is in the semi-flexed position (e.g. in a stumble or fall).

Ankle fractures

- Result predominantly from an inversion injury.
- Ligamentous injuries commonly occur in association with fractures, resulting in joint space widening.
- Ankle joint fractures are frequently seen only on one projection and so careful scrutiny of both views is required.
- Accessory ossicles below the medial and lateral malleoli are common and can be confused with fractures; ossicles have a well-corticated outline.
- Medial and lateral malleolus fractures – if both malleoli are broken, this is called a bimalleolar fracture and if the posterior portion of the talus is also fractured, this is called a trimalleolar.

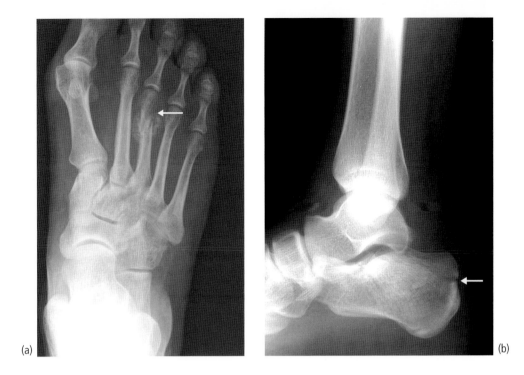

(a)

(b)

Figure 8.34 (a) Healing stress fracture of the third metatarsal (arrow); (b) calcaneal fracture (arrow).

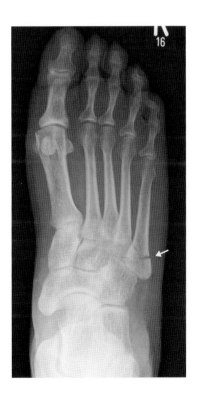

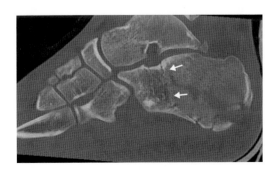

Figure 8.35 CT of calcaneal fracture affecting the articular surface.

Figure 8.36 Fifth metatarsal fracture (arrow).

Foot fractures

Calcaneal fracture

- Fractures are often bilateral and result from a twisting ankle injury or more commonly a fall from a height.
- May be confined to the calcaneum or extend to involve the subtalar or calcaneocuboid joints.
- Significant fractures – CT scanning for further evaluation and the need for surgical fixation.
- Associated fractures of the spine, pelvis, hips and knees may be present.

Talar fractures

- Falls onto the feet or violent dorsiflexion of the ankle may cause fractures to the anterior body or articular dome of the talus.
- Displaced fractures and dislocations often result in avascular necrosis.
- May require manipulation and/or open reduction and internal fixation.
- Dislocations of the talus require early reduction under general anaesthetic.

Fifth metatarsal fracture

- Ankle inversion injury may result in a fracture at the insertion of the peroneus brevis tendon – the base of the fifth metatarsal.
- Important not to misinterpret the normal unfused apophysis in children at the base of the fifth metatarsal as a fracture; the apophysis lies longitudinally whereas a fracture is transverse.

Metatarsal fractures and dislocations

- Multiple metatarsal fractures may be caused by heavy objects falling onto the feet or by a vehicle wheel.
- Tarsometatarsal (Lisfranc) dislocation: can be easily missed on standard foot X-rays. Check that the medial side of the second metatarsal is correctly aligned with the medial side of the middle cuneiform.

Stress fractures of the metatarsals

- Common: often caused by prolonged or unusual exercise ('March fracture'), but may occur without any obvious cause.
- Commonest site is the second metatarsal shaft, but the third metatarsal or rarely other metatarsals may be affected.
- X-rays are usually initially normal. Callus or periosteal reaction seen on after 2–3 weeks will confirm the diagnosis.
- Treatment is symptomatic with analgesia, elevation, rest and reduced activity as required.

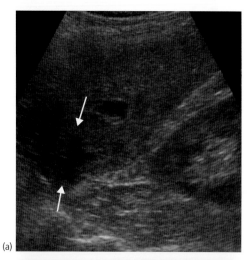

(a)

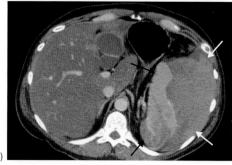

(b)

Figure 8.37 (a) Ultrasound of the spleen showing splenic haematoma (arrows); (b) CT abdomen with contrast enhancement – splenic rupture with haematoma (white arrows). Enhancing spleen (black arrows).

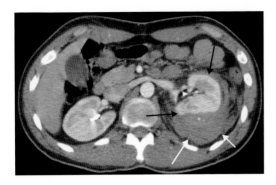

Figure 8.38 CT abdomen – contrast enhanced showing renal haematoma (white arrows) and kidney (black arrows).

Blunt abdominal trauma

Direct trauma to the abdomen may result in injuries to the underlying organs and is often the result of a car collision. The liver and spleen are the most frequently injured organs often associated with fractured ribs.

The primary mechanisms of injury are as follows.

- Compression force trauma.
- Deceleration force trauma, which classically causes hepatic tears and intimal injuries to the renal arteries.

Injuries to the spleen, liver, kidney, bowel and pancreas should be evaluated.

- Spleen – the most commonly injured organ in blunt trauma. Delayed complications may result from rupture of a subcapsular haematoma. Small lacerations can be managed by observation. Large lacerations need oversewing or splenectomy.
- Liver – lacerations and haematoma formation.
- Kidney – injury is common with falls or car accidents. A lacerated kidney will show contrast extravasation.
- Bowel – more commonly affected in penetrating trauma. Free air seen on plain films.

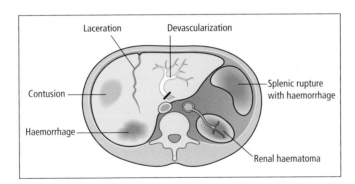

Figure 8.39 Blunt abdominal trauma.

Key point

Any patient with tachycardia or hypotension associated with left upper quadrant tenderness is assumed to have a ruptured spleen until proven otherwise

9

Paediatrics

'Children are not just small adults' is a well-worn phrase and applies in paediatric radiology too, where the different imaging modalities are used to help diagnose certain diseases that are only seen in children. Below are some of the commonly encountered conditions which will be helpful to the medical students of today and doctors of tomorrow.

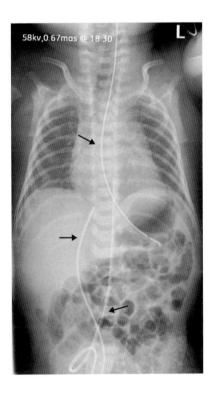

Figure 9.1 Premature neonate with nasogastric tube (top arrow), umbilical venous (middle arrow) and umbilical arterial (lower arrow) catheters.

Paediatric/Neonatal support tubing and lines

Neonates and children may need to have various tubes and lines inserted to facilitate their treatment while in hospital and sometimes outside of hospital too.

It is important to have a basic knowledge of the commonly encountered support tubing and lines that are usually identifiable on plain radiographs.

- **Oxygen tubing**: used to administer oxygen; usually seen as a faint tube overlying the thorax on chest radiographs and attached to a mask.
- **Nasogastric tube**: used for giving feeds into the stomach and also sometimes to drain the stomach; correct positioning is vital and if incorrectly placed, this can be fatal. Should be seen passing down the central mediastinum, crossing the carina or left main bronchus and then going into the left upper abdomen with tip beneath the left hemidiaphragm.
- **Endotracheal tube**: used to ventilate lungs of neonates and children; should be seen positioned within trachea and tip **above** level of the carina.
- **Umbilical venous catheter** (UVC): used to give medicines to neonates; inserted via the umbilicus into the umbilical vein, passing into the left portal vein, then through the ductus venosus into a hepatic vein and then the inferior vena cava and up to the right heart with the tip in the right cardiophrenic region. The tip should not be advanced into the right atrium as it can then stimulate the nerve fibres here and lead to arrhythmias.
- **Umbilical arterial catheter** (UAC): provides access to the arterial system for accurate measurement of arterial blood pressure, blood sampling and

Radiology: Lecture Notes, Fourth Edition. Pradip R. Patel.
© 2020 John Wiley & Sons Ltd. Published 2020 by John Wiley & Sons Ltd.
Companion website: www.wiley.com/go/patel/radiology

administration of intravascular fluids/medications; inserted via umbilical artery and into the aorta via the internal iliac artery. In order to avoid placement into the aortic branches (e.g. coeliac, mesenteric, renal arteries) and compromise blood supply to organs, it should be placed 'high' (T6 to T9 level) or 'low' (L3 to L5). The 'high' position is advisable as it leads to less vascular complications.

- **Percutaneous endoscopic gastrostomy** (PEG tube or feeding tube): used for feeding children with long-term impaired swallowing and at risk of aspiration; seen passing into the stomach and identifiable in the left upper abdomen on abdominal radiographs.

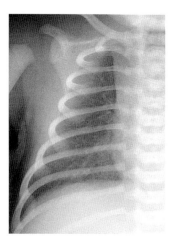 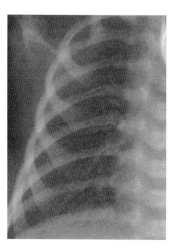 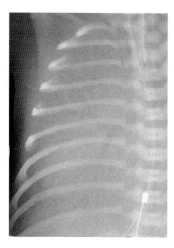

Figure 9.2 Normal neonatal chest progressing to mild and then severe hyaline membrane disease.

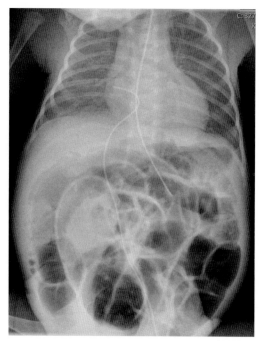

Figure 9.3 Abdomen radiograph in a premature neonate showing necrotising enterocolitis (dilated bowel with intramural gas) and hyaline membrane disease in the lung bases. The nasogastric tube is satisfactory; however, the longline is misplaced and needs to be pulled back, otherwise cardiac arrhythmias could occur.

Hyaline membrane disease

This is the most common cause of respiratory distress in premature births due to deficiency of pulmonary surfactant preventing alveolar distension. Transudation into the alveolar space and a lining of debris and dead cells (hyaline membrane) impair gaseous exchange and lead to hypoxia. The condition should be differentiated from meconium aspiration, neonatal pneumonia and congestive heart failure.

Radiological features

A chest X-ray may illustrate the following:

- typical ground glass or a fine granular appearance to the lungs;
- air bronchogram;
- low-volume lungs.

There is also usually a high chance of developing associated necrotising enterocolitis in the abdomen, which may be identified on plain radiography.

Complications

Usually from treatment by barotrauma from prolonged positive pressure ventilation, leading to pneumothorax; pneumomediastinum and pulmonary interstitial emphysema from overdistended alveoli leaking air.

Treatment

- Positive pressure ventilation to maintain patency of terminal alveoli and preserve oxygenation.
- Surfactant given via the endotracheal tube in ventilated babies.

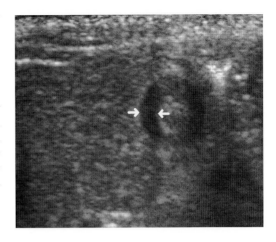

Figure 9.4 Pyloric stenosis: transverse ultrasound section of the pylorus with muscle thickening (arrows).

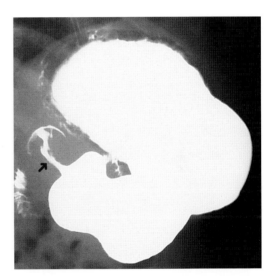

Figure 9.5 Pyloric stenosis: contrast examination of the stomach showing a narrowed elongated pyloric canal (arrow).

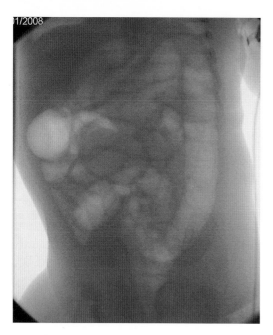

01/2008

Figure 9.6 Air enema reduction of the intussusception.

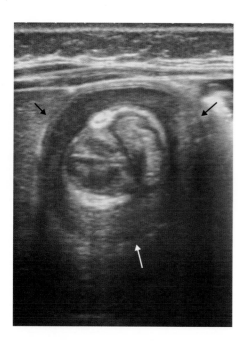

Figure 9.7 Ultrasound demonstrates the intussusception as a 'doughnut shaped' mass.

Pyloric stenosis

Pyloric stenosis is characterized by smooth muscle hypertrophy of the pyloric muscle. It usually presents between 3 and 6 weeks after birth, with a marked male : female preponderance in its incidence (4 : 1) and usually a positive family history of the condition. Pyloric stenosis is a clinical diagnosis, where the baby presents with projectile vomiting and the pyloric mass is often palpable clinically in the right upper quadrant of the abdomen ('olive-shaped mass'). In doubtful cases, an ultrasound or a water-soluble contrast meal is often diagnostic. Treatment is by correction of any electrolyte disturbance secondary to the vomiting and then a surgical myotomy of the pyloric muscle – Ramstedt's operation.

Presentation

- Vomiting (often projectile and not bile stained).
- Dehydration.
- Hypochloraemic alkalosis.
- Failure to thrive.

Radiological features

Ultrasound demonstrates the pyloric canal with the surrounding thickened muscle. *Water-soluble contrast examination* of the stomach can be performed in equivocal cases and shows delayed gastric emptying with elongation and narrowing of the pyloric canal.

Intussusception

An intussusception results from telescoping or invagination of one segment of bowel into another, causing mechanical obstruction. It is most common in the ileocaecal area where the terminal ileum invaginates into the caecum and ascending colon and may be palpable clinically as a mass in the right lower quadrant of the abdomen ('sausage-shaped mass'). Bowel infarction will ensue if left untreated.

Presentation

Occur most frequently in children up to 2 years of age: drowsiness; colicky abdominal pain; vomiting; blood per rectum ('redcurrent jelly stool'). Usually common in winter months as it is often associated with a preceding upper respiratory tract infection.

Radiological features

- Plain films may reveal a paucity of bowel gas in the right side of the abdomen, signs of small bowel obstruction and a soft tissue mass caused by the head of the intussusception.
- Ultrasound can usually identify the abdominal mass, which is seen as a 'doughnut' shaped structure.

Treatment

There is usually a high success rate for reduction of the intussusception with air enema or hydrostatic water enema. If this fails, surgical reduction is necessary.

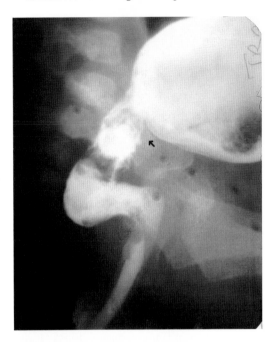

Figure 9.8 Hirschsprung's disease: barium enema showing the transition zone in the upper rectum (arrow).

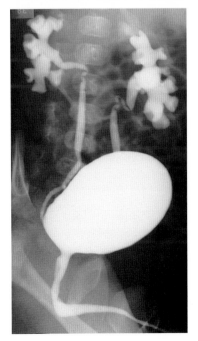

Figure 9.9 Micturating cystourethrogram (MCUG) showing gross bilateral vesico-ureteric reflux as the child is micturating.

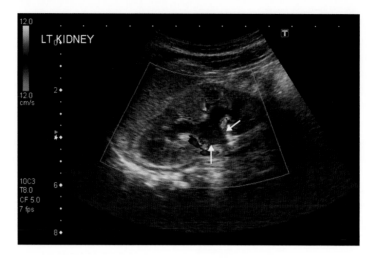

Figure 9.10 Ultrasound scan showing renal pelvis dilatation.

Hirschsprung's disease

In Hirschsprung's disease, an aganglionic segment of colon with a deficiency or absence of the myenteric plexus results in a non-distensible section, the proximal large bowel dilating and eventually resulting in a 'megacolon'. Rarely, aganglionosis may affect the whole of the large bowel. Diagnosis is by a rectal suction biopsy. Complications include necrotizing enterocolitis and caecal perforation secondary to bowel distension and ischaemia.

Presentation

- Failure to pass meconium within 24 hours, with signs of intestinal obstruction: abdominal distension and vomiting.
- Constipation dating from birth; presentation may be in infancy or in later life.

Radiological features

Plain abdominal films reveal a grossly dilated redundant colon loaded with faecal residue. On contrast enema examination, the involved segment is usually of a normal calibre (transition zone) but appears narrow, due to the distended colon above. Retention of contrast for up to 48 hours after the examination is a typical feature.

Vesico-ureteric reflux

The normal vesico-ureteric junction does not allow backward flow of urine from the bladder into the ureter. With reflux, the junction is incompetent and urine flows retrogradely up the ureters, especially during micturition. Reflux tends to be commonest in infancy and tends to resolve spontaneously during childhood, but is important to recognize because it can lead to recurrent urinary tract infection and chronic renal scarring may result. Urinary tract infection needs to be controlled in the presence of reflux, in order to prevent retardation of renal growth.

Radiological features

With severe reflux, ultrasound, micturating cystourethrography and isotope scanning may reveal the following:

- upper urinary tract dilatation;
- renal atrophy;
- renal scarring with loss of cortical tissue, especially at the upper pole.

Treatment

- Low-dose antibiotics to maintain a sterile urine and allow steady renal growth and development.
- Surgical correction in difficult cases.

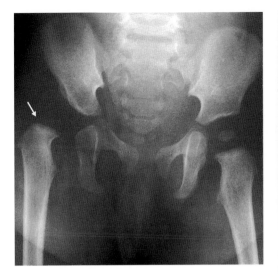

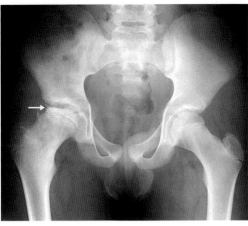

Figure 9.13 Perthes disease: flattening and increased density of the right femoral head (arrow).

Figure 9.11 Dislocation of the right hip on ultrasound (suitable before 6 months age). Plain radiograph (suitable after 6 months age) shows there is a delay in the appearance of the ossification centre of the head (arrow).

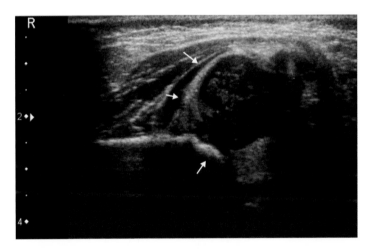

Figure 9.12 Ultrasound of the hip showing dislocation of the femoral head (upper arrows) outside the acetabulum (lower arrow).

Developmental dysplasia of the hips (DDH)

Developmental dysplasia of the hips more commonly affects females. Numerous factors may play a part in the aetiology of this condition, including genetic causes and breech presentation.

Radiological investigations

Ultrasound: useful below 6 months age.
Pelvis radiograph: useful after 6 months age.

Radiological features

At birth, films of the pelvis are of little help as the femoral head is not ossified. Ultrasound may demonstrate a shallow acetabulum and determine its slope; it visualizes the position of the femoral head, and any subluxation or dislocation. Ultrasound can also monitor treatment ensuring that the hip remains stable.

Plain films are more useful at a later stage, when there is ossification of the femoral head nucleus. Features to note are a delayed appearance of the ossific nucleus, a shallow acetabulum and displacement of the femoral head upwards and laterally from its normal position.

Perthes disease

Perthes disease is an osteonecrosis (osteochondritis) of the epiphysis of the femoral head likely to be due to a deficient blood supply. It is five times common in males, with a peak incidence at 4–8 years and 10% of cases may be bilateral. Hip pain and limp are the main presenting features. Trauma and previous surgical reduction of a congenital dislocation of the hip are aetiological factors.

Radiological features

The following appearances may be seen in the femoral head on plain films:

- reduction in size;
- increased density;
- fragmentation and condensation;
- persistent deformity after healing with associated thickening of the femoral neck.
- MRI can detect avascular necrosis earlier than plain films and may be useful to assess progress and treatment.

Complications

Increased risk of degenerative disease in adulthood, leading to pain, osteoarthritis and consideration for an early hip replacement.

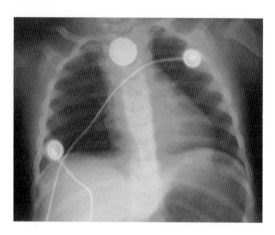

Figure 9.15 Chest radiographs showing swallowed coin. ECG leads are in position.

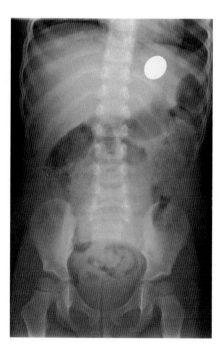

Figure 9.16 Swallowed coin in the upper abdomen.

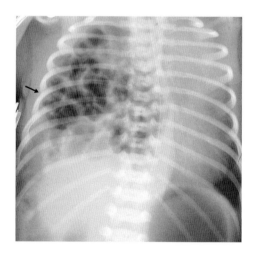

Figure 9.14 Congenital diaphragmatic hernia: multiple bowel loops in the right thorax (arrow).

Congenital diaphragmatic hernia

A congenital defect in the diaphragm, more common on the left, allows bowel protrusion into the thoracic cavity and usually results in respiratory distress. Herniation may occur at three sites, though those causing neonatal respiratory distress are usually of the Bochdalek type.

- Foramen of Bochdalek: posterior diaphragm.
- Foramen of Morgagni: anterior diaphragm.
- Oesophageal hiatus.

The main differential diagnosis for this condition is congenital cystic adenomatoid malformation (CCAM).

Radiological features

Antenatal ultrasound examination often detects the herniation. A chest X-ray illustrates either cyst-like changes or the typical appearance of multiple bowel loops in the thorax. Mediastinal shift is away from the affected side. Abdominal films may show the absence or paucity of bowel loops, as these have herniated into the affected side of the chest.

Treatment

This is a neonatal surgical emergency as it can seriously affect the baby's breathing; therefore, urgent surgical repair of the diaphragm is required, but because the associated lung in the affected hemithorax is hypoplastic, it can lead to pulmonary hypertension and cause significant mortality.

Swallowed foreign bodies

Children exploring their surrounding world will put any object into their mouths and will then often unintentionally swallow it.

The peak incidence is between 6 months and 6 years.

The commonest objects are coins; however, anything that can fit into a child's mouth can end up being swallowed. Some modern toys have button batteries and if these are swallowed, then urgent referral to a paediatric surgeon is necessary as these can set up electrical currents across body tissues and lead to complications such as bowel perforation.

Usually, radiographs of the chest and abdomen are done; however, the neck may also be included where necessary.

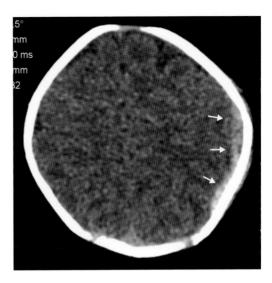

Figure 9.17 CT head in a baby showing a subtle left subdural haematoma (arrow): 'shaken baby syndrome'.

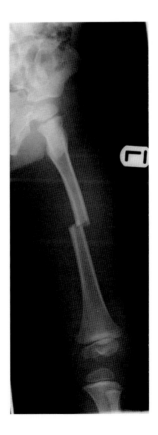

Figure 9.18 Radiograph of fractured femur in a child.

Non-accidental injury

Doctors and all those who come into contact with children and families in their everyday work and in situations outside of their work have a duty to safeguard and promote the welfare of children.

Non-accidental injury is when a child suffers physical and/or psychological abuse in the hands of their carers or others involved in their everyday life and this should be recognized and acted on immediately, to safeguard the child from further harm.

There is a usually a safeguarding lead and team in every hospital and when alerted of a potential case, they follow certain protocols to ensure that the child is kept in a 'place of safety' until the matter is investigated and resolved fully.

As medical students, it is important to have a basic understanding of non-accidental injury and its radiology.

Presentation

- non-accidental injury may be suspected on the basis of unexplained injuries, injuries more severe than expected from the history, injuries of different ages;
- usually common under 2 years old (smaller children cannot protect themselves from their bigger perpetrators);
- there may be presentation with collapse or near-miss cot death due to cerebral injury;
- there may be multiple injuries with presentation to different hospitals and delayed presentation;
- non-accidental injury has many different 'faces' and as doctors, we should remain vigilant.

Radiological investigations

- Imaging should always include skeletal survey in children under two years old and skeletal survey and CT head scan in children under one year old.
- Children who are older than one year and have external evidence of head trauma and/or abnormal neurological symptoms or signs should also have a CT head scan.

Radiological features

- head: skull fractures, facial fractures, intracranial bleed (subdural haematoma);
- neck/spine: cervical spine injury, haematomas, vertebral fractures;
- chest: rib fractures, clavicle fractures, medistinal injury, haemothorax;
- abdomen: liver/spleen injury, bowel tears, intra-abdominal bleeding;
- upper/lower limbs: spiral fractures, metaphyseal corner fractures ('bucket handle tears');
- hands/feet: fractures and dislocations.

10

Obstetrics and gynaecology

Investigations

Plain films

An incidental finding from plain films may diagnose calcifications in an ovarian dermoid or calcification in uterine fibroids.

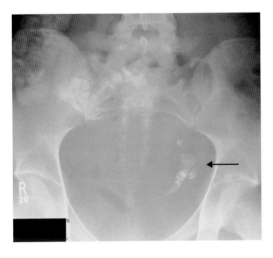

Figure 10.1 Plain film of the pelvis showing an ovarian dermoid with calcification and teeth (arrow).

Ultrasound

This is the principal imaging modality and can safely monitor pregnancy, from early gestation to term pregnancy. It is useful to confirm the presence of a viable early gestation, in the detection of ectopic pregnancy, the position of the placenta and fetal anomalies; it will assist in amniocentesis to make it a relatively safe procedure.

The uterus and ovaries are well visualized by a pelvic ultrasound scan. A more precise and detailed examination is obtained using a transvaginal probe.

- Uterus: ultrasound assesses size, outline, position and myometrial abnormalities such as leiomyomas and congenital uterine anomalies.
- Endometrium: this is seen as an echogenic linear area, the appearances varying through the menstrual cycle. It is poorly visualized in postmenopausal women due to atrophic changes and carcinoma may be suspected when there is abnormal thickening or configuration.
- Endometrial cavity: ultrasound accurately delineates retained products of conception and may visualize polyps.
- Fallopian tubes: generally not adequately seen, unless there is a hydrosalpinx.
- Ovaries: appear as oval structures lateral to the uterus, being small and atrophic in postmenopausal women. Follicular development can be monitored using ultrasound.
- Adnexae, cul-de-sac: detection of masses and free fluid.

Radiology: Lecture Notes, Fourth Edition. Pradip R. Patel.
© 2020 John Wiley & Sons Ltd. Published 2020 by John Wiley & Sons Ltd.
Companion website: www.wiley.com/go/patel/radiology

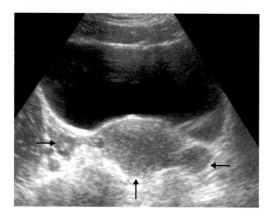

Figure 10.2 Normal uterus (arrow ↑) and ovaries (arrows → ←).

Hysterosalpingography

This is carried out by direct injection of the contrast into the cervical canal to assess the uterine cavity, any congenital abnormalities and check the patency of the fallopian tubes.

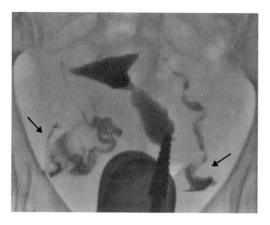

Figure 10.3 Normal hysterosalpingogram showing patient fallopian tubes with bilateral peritoneal spill (arrows).

Computed tomography (CT)

This is valuable in the staging of pelvic neoplasms and determines local spread as well as associated pelvic or para-aortic lymphadenopathy and liver metastases.

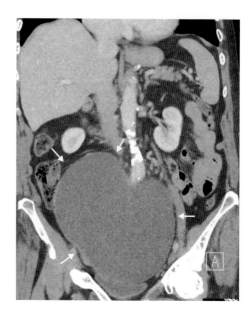

Figure 10.4 Coronal CT reconstruction showing a large ovarian cyst (arrows).

Magnetic resonance imaging (MRI)

Useful in the evaluation of fibroids and pelvic malignancy, and in imaging the fetus and placenta, due to the absence of ionizing radiation and the high soft tissue contrast resolution.

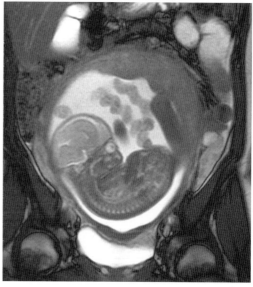

Figure 10.5 MRI of a normal fetus.

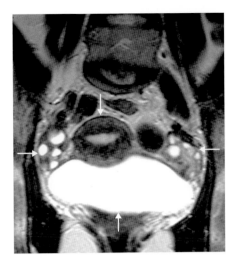

Figure 10.6 MRI pelvis showing a normal uterus (arrow ↓), bladder (arrow ↑) and bilateral polycystic ovaries (arrows → ←).

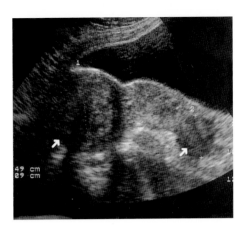

Figure 10.8 MRI: T1 and T2 sequences showing uterine fibroids (arrows).

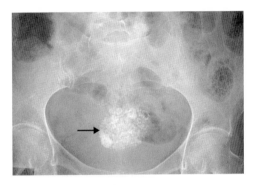

Figure 10.9 Calcification in a fibroid (arrow).

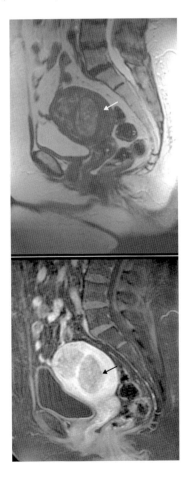

Figure 10.7 Ultrasound examination demonstrating two large fibroids (arrows) in the uterus.

Uterine fibroids (leiomyoma)

Fibroids are common tumours resulting from benign overgrowth of smooth muscle and connective tissue and occur in up to 50% of women over the age of 30. Fibroids generally shrink after the menopause.

Radiological features

The following may be noted on ultrasound.

- Calcification: also shown on plain films and CT.
- Enlarged uterus, with a distorted outline.
- Lobular or round masses of variable echogenicity being intramural, subserosal or submucousal.

MRI is more sensitive at detecting fibroids than ultrasound.

Complications

- Infertility.
- Dystocia.
- Malignant sarcomatous degeneration (rare).
- Cystic degeneration.

Treatment

- Myomectomy.
- Uterine artery embolization of fibroids.

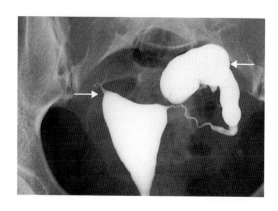

Figure 10.12 Hysterosalpingography: occlusion of the right fallopian tube (arrow →) and a left hydrosalpinx (arrow ←).

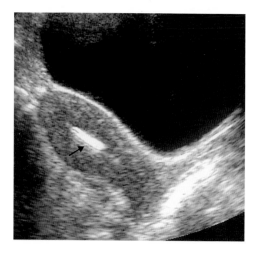

Figure 10.10 Ultrasound: IUCD in the endometrial cavity (arrows).

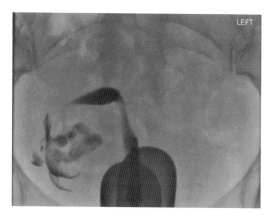

Figure 10.13 Hysterosalpingogram showing normal right fallopian tube and a left salpingectomy for an ectopic pregnancy.

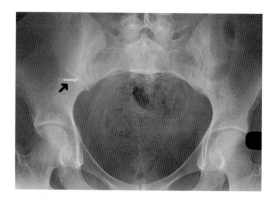

Figure 10.11 Perforation with IUCD seen lying over the right iliac bone (arrow).

Intrauterine contraceptive device

- Ultrasound accurately assesses the position of an intrauterine contraceptive device (IUCD), identified lying in the endometrial cavity as a linear echogenic structure.
- The commonest cause of non-visualization is expulsion of the device.
- A plain abdominal film is recommended, as the IUCD may have perforated through the myometrium and be lying free in the abdominal cavity.
- Perforation is usually silent without symptoms and the IUCD can be removed by laparoscopy.

Fallopian tube occlusion

- Causes of occluded fallopian tubes include previous infection, peritonitis (especially from appendicitis) or tubal surgery.
- Radiological confirmation can be obtained by hysterosalpingography, the injection of iodinated contrast into the uterine cavity to assess the uterus and patency of fallopian tubes, which is seen with X-ray. HyCoSy is a similar method, but uses injection of ultrasound contrast and transvaginal ultrasound. Usually, there is rapid filling of the fallopian tubes with free spillage of contrast into the peritoneal cavity, confirming tubal patency.

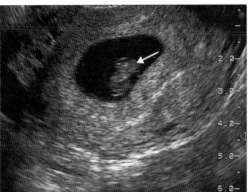

Figure 10.14 Gestation at 6 weeks (arrow).

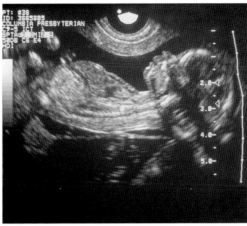

Figure 10.15 Gestation at 16 weeks.

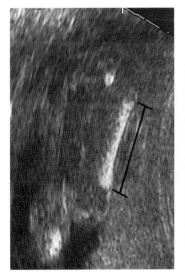
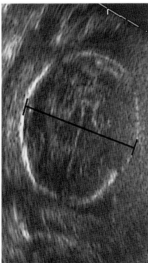
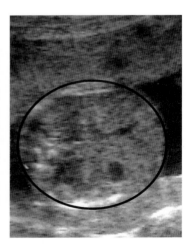

Figure 10.16 Fetal measurements on ultrasound: femur length, biparietal diameter and abdominal circumference.

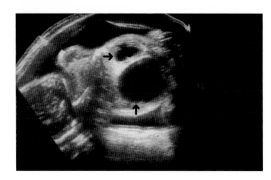

Figure 10.17 Ultrasound demonstrating a distended fetal bladder (↑) with a hydronephrotic kidney (→).

Fetal anomaly

A vast number of fetal abnormalities can be detected by ultrasound, some of which include:

- central nervous system: anencephaly, spina bifida, meningocoele, encephalocoele and hydrocephalus;
- chest: cardiac anomalies and pulmonary hypoplasia;
- gastrointestinal tract: duodenal atresia;
- renal tract: hydronephrosis, polycystic disease;
- skeletal: dwarfism.

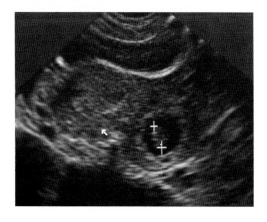

Figure 10.18 Ectopic pregnancy: the gestation sac (between ++) is seen outside the uterus (arrow).

Gestation: 6 weeks

- Ultrasound can be performed to confirm and date pregnancy or to detect complications such as an ectopic pregnancy or threatened abortion.
- The earliest detection of the sac is at 5–6 weeks on a pelvic ultrasound scan, seen as a ring-shaped echo-free area in the uterine cavity.
- Gestation age can be estimated by sac volume and the fetal crown–rump length; fetal cardiac pulsation is visible at approximately 7 weeks.
- Transvaginal scanning produces a more detailed evaluation – gestation sac and cardiac pulsation are recognized earlier than with a transabdominal scan.

Gestation: 11–13 weeks

Ultrasound assesses gestation age, fetal viability and fetal abnormalities.

Nuchal translucency (measurement of the normal fluid-filled subcutaneous space identified at the back of the fetal neck) is used in conjunction with serum markers for screening for chromosomal abnormalities.

The placenta can be evaluated for its location and any accompanying abnormalities.

Fetal parameters utilized for gestation age are:

- biparietal diameter;
- head circumference;
- abdominal circumference;
- femur length.

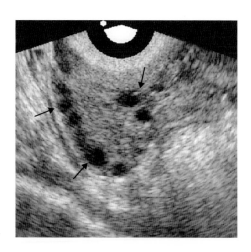

Figure 10.19 Polycystic ovary: transvaginal scan demonstrating an enlarged ovary with multiple small cysts (arrows).

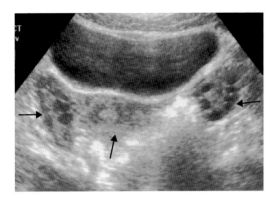

Figure 10.20 Transabdominal scan showing enlarged polycystic ovaries (arrows →←). Compare with the size of the uterus (arrow ↑).

Ectopic gestation

Ectopic pregnancy arises from failure of a fertilized ovum to reach the uterine cavity with subsequent implantation in the fallopian tube. Rarely, implantation may occur in the ovary or peritoneal cavity. An increased risk of ectopic pregnancy exists with pelvic inflammatory disease, use of an IUCD and a previous history of tubal surgery or ectopic gestation.

Radiological features

A normal ultrasound examination does not exclude an ectopic pregnancy, evaluation being more precise using transvaginal scanning. Some of the features below may be present:

- absence of gestation sac in uterine cavity (with positive pregnancy test);
- visualization of gestation sac or fetus outside the uterine cavity;
- endometrial thickening;
- free pelvic fluid;
- adnexal mass.

The tubal pregnancy often ceases at 6–10 weeks either by tubal rupture or tubal abortion.

Polycystic ovaries

- Polycystic ovaries are associated with chronic anovulation due to disturbances of luteinizing hormone (LH) and follicle stimulating hormone (FSH).
- The classical clinical features that suggest polycystic ovary syndrome (PCOS) are obesity, hirsutism, infertility and oligomenorrhoea (Stein–Leventhal syndrome). However, many women have biochemical abnormalities without these features and present with menstrual irregularity.
- Ultrasound features of PCOS include ovarian enlargement of greater than 10 mls and/or more than 12 follicles between 2–9 mm.

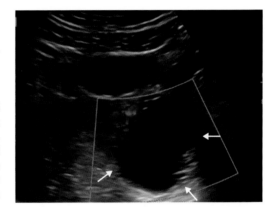

Figure 10.21 Benign ovarian cyst: thin-walled simple cystic structure (arrow) with abscent Doppler signal on colour flow indicating no vascularity.

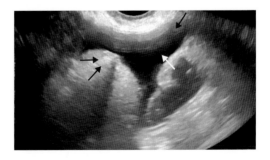

Figure 10.22 Dermoid cyst: transvaginal ultrasound demonstrating echogenic (fat) components (black arrows) as well as fluid (white arrow).

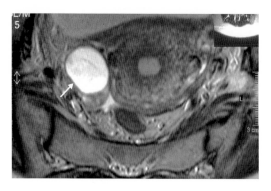

Figure 10.23 MRI pelvis: simple right ovarian cyst (arrow).

Benign ovarian cyst

Ovarian cysts are common and can attain sizes that can occupy most of the abdominal cavity.

Radiological features

On ultrasound, the typical appearances indicating a benign lesion are: thin walls; free of internal echoes; lack of internal septations.

Simple cysts <6 cm should have a follow-up ultrasound. A large cyst may show on a plain abdominal film as a soft tissue mass arising out of the pelvis. Complex cysts may be haemorrhagic or endometrioma.

MRI is a very useful modality to characterize indeterminate lesions on ultrasound and can detect the presence of blood in endometriomas, fat in dermoid cysts and enhancing tissue in malignant or borderline lesions.

Types of common benign cysts

- Follicular cysts. These are unruptured graafian follicles. They resolve spontaneously and generally do not attain a size >6 cm. Serial scans confirm resolution of these cysts.
- Corpus luteum cysts. The corpus luteum normally degenerates after ovulation, but may persist, sometimes with internal haemorrhage.
- Mucinous cystadenoma and serous cystadenoma are benign cysts with a malignant potential, a far more frequent occurrence in the latter.
- Endometriomas. Endometriosis within the ovaries results in the formation of blood-filled 'chocolate cysts', which may demonstrate solid tissue representing clot.
- Dermoid cysts. Benign dermoid cysts are also known as mature cystic teratoma. Classically they contain sebum and/or hair, appearing very echogenic, but with marked posterior shadowing. This results in the 'tip of the iceberg sign', meaning that only a small part of the cyst may be visible.

Complications

- Torsion: twisting on its pedicle interrupts the blood supply, initially venous then arterial. Results in severe pain when this complication arises.
- Infection.
- Rupture: pain and vomiting.
- Haemorrhage into cyst.

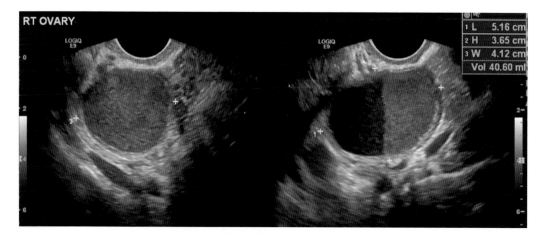

Figure 10.24 Endometrioma: transvaginal ultrasound demonstrating a unilocular cystic lesion with layering ground glass echoes indicating haemorrhage of different ages.

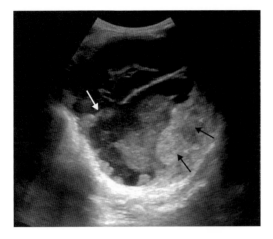

Figure 10.25 Transvaginal ultrasound demonstrating malignant serous cystadenocarcinoma. There is irregular solid tumour (black arrow) as well as complex irregular septation (white arrow).

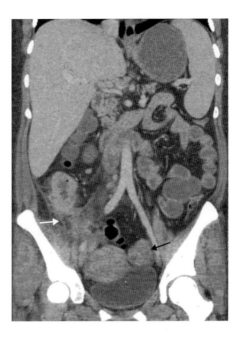

Figure 10.27 Coronal CT demonstrates caecal carcinoma (white arrow) with metastasis to the left ovary (black arrow).

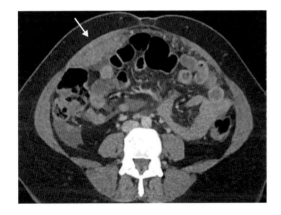

Figure 10.26 Staging CT demonstrates omental metastases from ovarian carcinoma (arrow).

Ovarian carcinoma

Ovarian carcinoma is the commonest cause of death from female genital tract cancer.

Presentation

- Asymptomatic discovery on routine examination.
- Ascites and/or pelvic mass.
- Persistent abdominal distension (bloating).
- Early satiety/loss of appetite.
- Pelvic or abdominal pain.
- Increased urinary urgency and/or frequency.

Radiological investigations

- Ultrasound.
- CT for staging.
- MRI may be useful in assessing likelihood of malignancy when the lesion is indeterminate on ultrasound.

Radiological features

- Ultrasound is the most appropriate initial investigation and the diagnosis can frequently be made by this technique. Malignancy may be suspected in a pelvic mass if the following features are present: thick irregular septations with nodules; thick wall with irregularity of the inner wall; mixed solid and cystic components; local invasion; ascites (although this may also be seen in benign lesions); peritoneal and lymph node metastases.
- CT is essential in staging the tumour prior to resection.
- Malignant ovarian tumours.
- Malignant cystadenocarcinoma.
- Metastases: Krukenberg secondaries from mucus-secreting stomach or colon carcinoma.
- Non-epithelial tumours such as granulosa cell, theca cell, androblastoma, dysgerminoma, malignant teratoma.

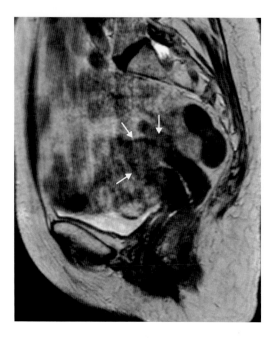

Figure 10.29 MRI image demonstrating a carcinoma in the superior endometrium (arrow).

Endometrial carcinoma

This is the fourth most common cancer in women and has significantly increased in incidence due to factors such as obesity, tamoxifen and a reduction in the rate of hysterectomy.

Presentation

- Postmenopausal bleeding.
- Abnormal bleeding in premenopausal patients.
- Vaginal discharge.
- Abnormal smear.

Radiological investigations

- Ultrasound.
- MRI pelvis.
- CT chest, abdomen and pelvis.

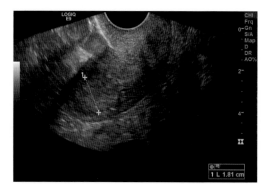

Figure 10.28 Endometrial carcinoma: transvaginal ultrasound demonstrating a markedly thickened endometrium (between ++). A normal postmenopausal endometrium should not usually measure more than 4 mm.

Radiological features

- Transvaginal ultrasound is the initial investigation and usually demonstrates a thickened endometrium in a postmenopausal patient (>4 mm). The endometrium may demonstrate vascularity on colour flow Doppler. Ultrasound is not helpful in patients taking tamoxifen as this often makes the endometrium appear thickened and cystic. All patients with persistent postmenopausal bleeding or discharge should have an endometrial biopsy.

- MRI is used for local staging to determine whether the cancer has penetrated the deep myometrium or extends beyond the uterus.
- CT is used to stage for distant metastases beyond the pelvis.

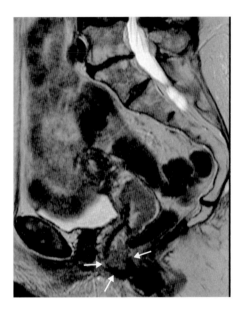

Figure 10.30 MRI image showing a large tumour in the cervix (arrow).

Cervical carcinoma

Cervical carcinoma is the third most common gynaecological malignancy and is related to infection from Human Papilloma Virus.

Presentation

- Abnormal cervical screening smear.
- Vaginal bleeding.
- Vaginal discharge.
- Dyspareunia/pelvic pain.

Radiological investigations

- MRI.
- CT.
- PET CT.

Radiological features

- MRI is used for local staging to assess the tumour size and detect whether the tumour has spread beyond the cervix, e.g. into the lower vagina or parametrium. Endovaginal MRI is useful in smaller tumours where fertility-preserving surgery (trachelectomy) is being considered.
- CT is used to stage for distant metastatic disease and complications such as hydronephrosis.
- PET CT provides more accurate staging than CT alone.

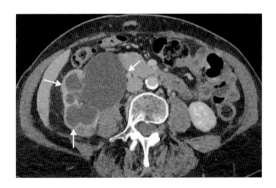

Figure 10.31 CT showing right hydronephrosis secondary to right ureteric obstruction from a large cervical carcinoma (arrows).

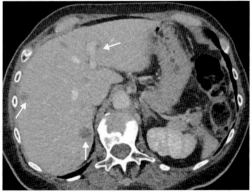

Figure 10.32 CT image showing multiple liver metastases from cervical carcinoma (arrows).

11

Neuroradiology

Neuroradiology: investigations

Plain films

The need for plain skull films in diagnosis has virtually disappeared now mainly used after surgery to evaluate hardware.

Plain spine films are routinely used in the context of trauma allowing quick evaluation of the skeleton.

Ultrasound

In adults, ultrasound is mainly used for imaging of the extracranial vascular structures. In particular, it is used as the first-line investigation for carotid artery stenosis. It provides anatomical assessment of the vessel wall and when utilizing the Doppler effect, it is able to look for blood flow velocity.

The neonatal brain can also be imaged with ultrasound by using the open anterior fontanelle as a window for sound waves to travel into the brain. This technique allows rapid assessment of the neonatal brain to assess for intraventricular haemorrhage, hydrocephalus or other suspected intracranial pathology.

Computed tomography (CT)

CT data are acquired rapidly, in the order of seconds and minutes. This makes CT a highly valuable tool in acute trauma and unwell patients.

CT is also especially useful in the assessment of bones for the assessment of the vertebrae and small bones within the skull base.

Magnetic resonance imaging (MRI)

MRI utilizes the properties of hydrogen atoms and its reaction to an external stimulus (radio-frequency) when placed in a high magnetic field environment. This creates a signal which allows subsequent generation of interpretable data.

MRI is therefore highly sensitive for the detection of water (or oedema). This property allows us to image the brain in exquisite detail and to detect pathology by looking at altered brain anatomy and brain water context.

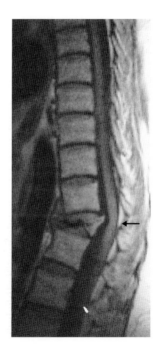

Figure 11.1 MRI: vertebral collapse of T12 causing early spinal cord compression (arrow).

Radiology: Lecture Notes, Fourth Edition. Pradip R. Patel.
© 2020 John Wiley & Sons Ltd. Published 2020 by John Wiley & Sons Ltd.
Companion website: www.wiley.com/go/patel/radiology

There is a growing interest and use of functional MRI in clinical practice. Instead of purely looking at anatomical detail, MRI can be used to look at brain physiology. Diffusion-weighted MRI is currently the most widely used technique and employs the assessment of water movement within structures. It is now routinely used in imaging strokes and brain ischemia. Functional MRI looking at blood flow is increasingly used as a surrogate for brain activity. This technique has allowed a greater understanding of brain function in emotion, behaviour and reasoning.

Arteriography

Arteriography is useful in evaluation of the intracranial vessels and has made it possible to treat certain brain conditions using minimally invasive techniques. Arteries of the cerebral circulation may be visualized by contrast injection into the aortic arch or selectively into the carotid and vertebral arteries.

Nuclear medicine

Using radio isotopes as tracers for brain imaging is now common practice. Detection of areas of accumulation and patterns of accumulation provides insight into brain function and the diagnosis of brain disease. Accurate diagnosis of Parkinson's disease can be made using dopamine markers. Alzheimer's and other neurodegenerative disease can be imaged with this technique using glucose metabolism or specific markers.

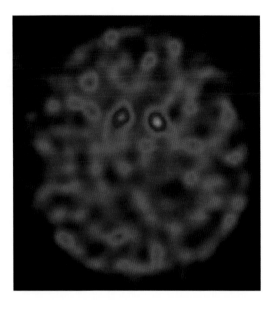

Figure 11.2 Brain Ioflupane DaTSCAN showing reduced tracer uptake throughout the stiata consistent with Parkinson's syndrome.

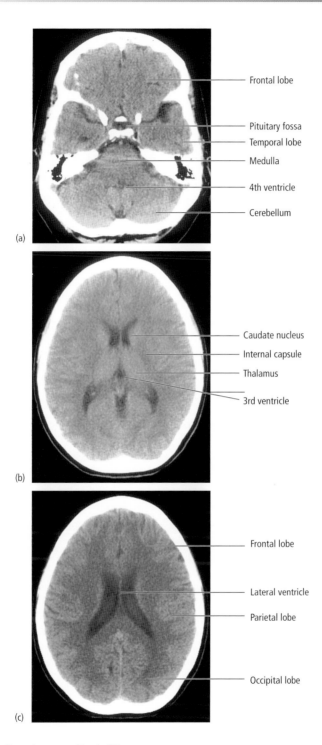

Frontal lobe

Pituitary fossa

Temporal lobe

Medulla

4th ventricle

Cerebellum

(a)

Caudate nucleus

Internal capsule

Thalamus

3rd ventricle

(b)

Frontal lobe

Lateral ventricle

Parietal lobe

Occipital lobe

(c)

Figure 11.3 Sections through a normal brain CT.

Normal brain CT

Data obtained from CT are depicted on a grey scale. High-density material (those that absorb greater proportion of radiation, for instance bone) is depicted closer to white while low density material (for instance water or fat) is depicted as closer to black. This is termed the Hounsfield unit.

A CT study can be examined quickly using the principle of comparing the two sides for asymmetry in combination with a detailed knowledge of normal anatomy. Special attention is paid to:

- midline shift;
- localized area of altered density;
- presence of mass lesion.

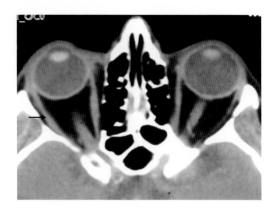

Figure 11.5 CT through normal orbits showing optic nerve (←) and the lateral rectus muscle (→).

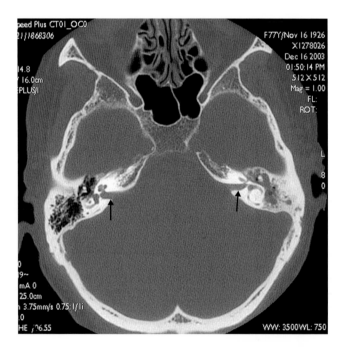

Figure 11.4 CT through normal petrous bone showing the internal auditory canals (arrows).

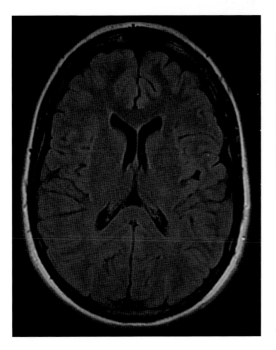

Figure 11.6 Axial FLAIR through the lateral ventricles and the region of the internal capsule; note the CSF appears black as the effect of water has been nullified to improve conspicuity of brain lesion.

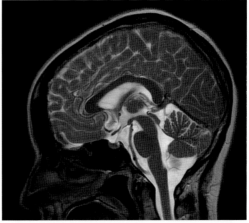

Figure 11.8 Section through a normal brain MRI scan.

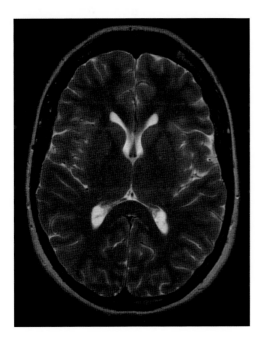

Figure 11.7 Axial T2 scan; the CSF appears white.

Normal brain MRI

MRI is the most sensitive imaging modality for the diagnosis of intracranial pathology. Anatomy is delineated in exquisite detail, more accurately than CT. Vascular anatomy can also be visualized without the aid of intravenous contrast.

The main disadvantages are the need for greater patient cooperation, as examination times are longer than for CT, typically in the order of 20–30 minutes for a brain MRI. Also, patients with ferromagnetic objects (e.g. certain types of implant, metallic foreign bodies, pacing wires) must be scanned with caution. There is the risk that these objects become magnetized and dislodge from the body when placed in the high magnetic field environment. This can have a catastrophic consequence.

MRI can be displayed in multiple projections and volumetric data can be easily manipulated. Unlike CT, the obtained data can be portrayed in several different ways depending on the type of pulse sequence used. The types of sequences used in MRI are complex and numerous and beyond the scope of this chapter.

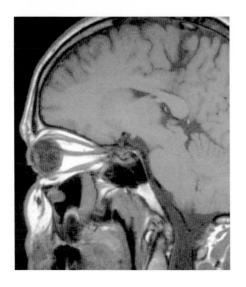

Figure 11.9 Sagittal MRI through the orbits.

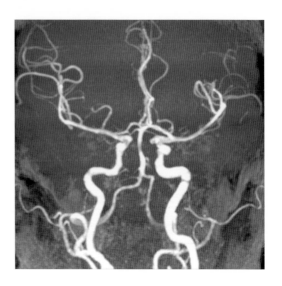

Figure 11.11 MRI scan of the intracranial arterial circulation, obtained without any administered contrast using a time of flight technique.

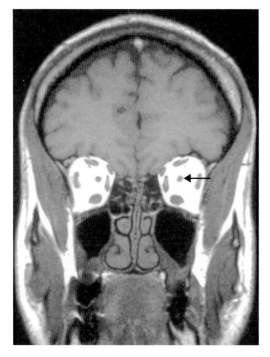

Figure 11.10 Coronal scan through the orbits. Note the central optic nerve (arrow) surrounded by the ocular muscles.

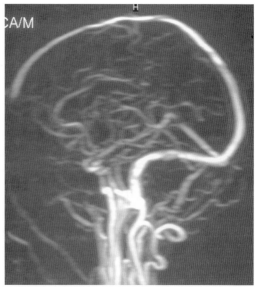

Figure 11.12 Sagittal MRI scan of the venous circulation.

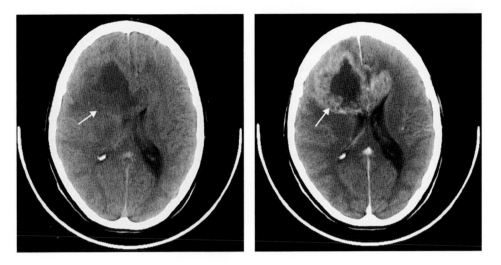

Figure 11.13 Glioma: CT scan pre- and post-contrast showing a large frontal mass (arrows).

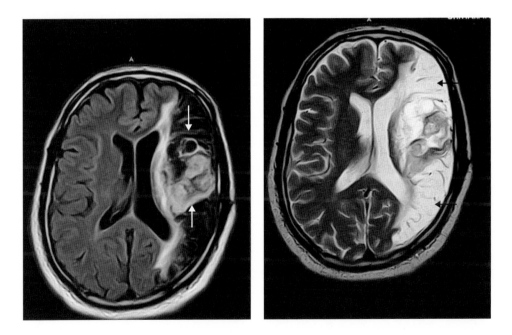

Figure 11.14 T1 and T2 MRI showing a large parietal lobe glioma (↑↓) with the T2 sequence showing extensive oedema around the tumour (white; ←).

Glioma

Primary brain tumours cause neurological symptoms due to distortion, pressure and displacement of adjacent structures. Gliomas are the commonest primary intracranial tumour.

Benign tumours can also cause a severe neurological deficit from the effect of expansion of the tumour in a confined space.

Radiological features

- Generally, plain films are no longer in use but may occasionally show calcification.
- On CT and MRI, the tumour appears as an area of altered density, with surrounding oedema and mass effect. Significant enhancement usually follows intravenous contrast.
- MRI is the investigation of choice, but CT is still widely utilized due to its availability.
- Low-grade gliomas – well-differentiated afford a better prognosis.
- High-grade gliomas – undifferentiated or anaplastic carry a worse prognosis.

Major types

- Astrocytoma – astrocytes.
- Oligodendroglioma – oligodendrocytes.
- Ependymoma – ependymal cells.

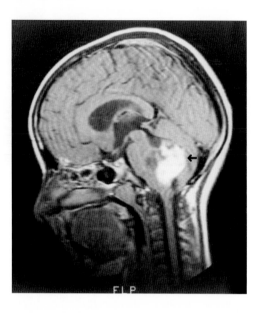

Figure 11.15 Astrocytoma: coronal MRI in a child with a posterior fossa mass (arrow).

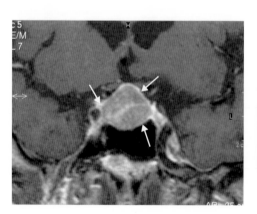
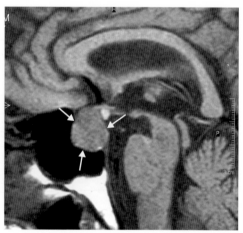

Figure 11.16 MRI: coronal section showing a large pituitary tumour enhancing after intravenous gadolinium (arrows). The sagittal T1 section demonstrates the tumour (arrows) in the pituitary fossa.

Posterior fossa tumour

The posterior fossa contains the cerebellum, pons and medulla oblongata. Up to 75% of intracranial tumours in children occur below the tentorium cerebelli in the posterior fossa.

Presentation

- Ataxia.
- Headache.
- Vomiting.
- Nystagmus.
- Cranial nerve dysfunction.

Tumour types

- Medulloblastoma.
- Ependymoma.
- Astrocytoma.

Pituitary tumour

- Pituitary adenomas are usually benign and only rarely undergo malignant change.
- Microadenoma <1 cm in diameter, or macroadenomas >1 cm.
- Prolactinoma is the most common pituitary tumour.
- Tumours are slow growing and penetrate adjacent structures.
- Presenting features depend on whether it is a hormone-secreting or deficiency tumour.

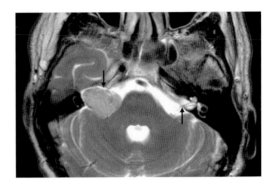

Figure 11.17 MRI showing a large acoustic neuroma at the right cerebello-pontine angle (↓). Note the normal 7th and 8th cranial nerves in the left auditory meatus (↑).

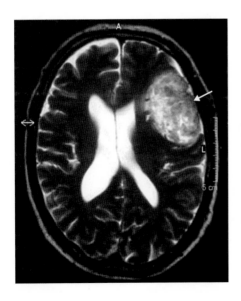

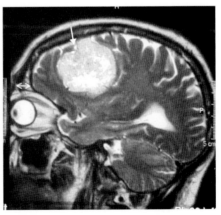

Figure 11.18 MRI brain; sagittal and axial scans showing a well-defined mass which is smooth in outline – meningioma (arrows).

Acoustic neuroma

Presentation

- Ipsilateral sensorineural hearing loss, balance disturbance, altered gait, tinnitus, vertigo, nausea, vomiting.
- MRI is the investigation of choice. Benign primary intracranial tumour from the myelin cells of the 8th nerve (vestibulocochlear).
- Grows into the internal auditory canal and extends into the posterior fossa.

Meningioma

Meningiomas are tumours that arise contiguously to the meninges. They represent 15–20% of primary brain tumours and are often discovered fortuitously when CT or MRI is done to assess for unrelated diseases or conditions.

- Benign, well-defined lesions arising from any part of the meningeal covering of the brain.
- Commonly found at the surface of the brain, either over the convexity or at the skull base.
- Frequent sites are the falx, parasagittal region and sphenoid wing.
- They usually grow slowly, and may produce severe morbidity before causing death.
- CT and MRI show well-defined lesions enhancing strongly and diffusely after intravenous contrast.

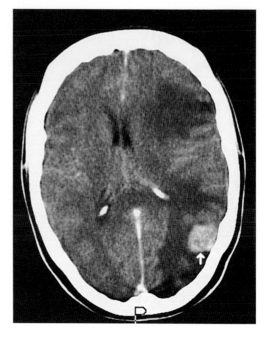

Figure 11.19 CT brain: metastasis enhancing after contrast; note the surrounding oedema (black).

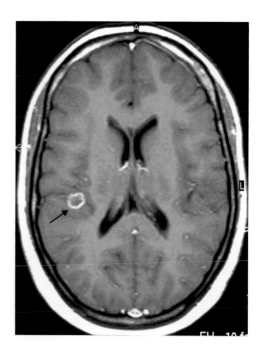

Figure 11.20 Small ring enhancing lesion in the right parietal lobe (arrow). The main differential lies between a secondary deposit and an abscess.

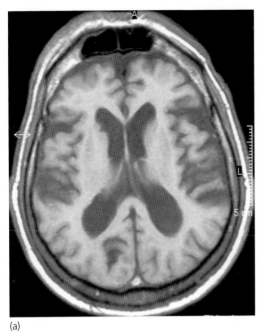

(a)

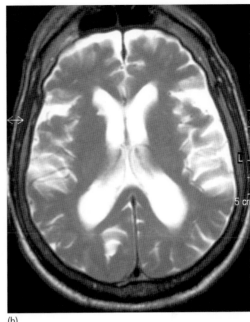

(b)

Figure 11.21 MRI showing cerebral atrophy. Note the volume loss with increased CSF space surrounding the brain (a) T1 CSF black and (b) T2 CSF white.

Cerebral metastases

Metastases are some of the commonest malignant cerebral lesions, involve any part of the brain and may be single or multiple. CT and MRI often cannot reliably distinguish between a primary neoplasm and a solitary secondary tumour, but the clinical setting may help. Multiple lesions are almost certainly metastases. Secondaries to the brain are commonly from bronchial, breast and gastrointestinal neoplasms.

Radiological features

Metastases can be haemorrhagic, cystic or calcified and they may cavitate; surrounding oedema is invariably present. After intravenous contrast, CT almost always shows enhancement of either the whole lesion or around the periphery, due to breakdown of the blood–brain barrier.

Treatment

- Palliative: dexamethasone reduces oedema and relieves headache; radiotherapy.
- Surgical resection occasionally for a solitary metastasis.

Cerebral atrophy

Atrophic changes in the brain are usually idiopathic. Causes include:

- degenerative conditions;
- trauma;
- drugs;
- infection (end stage);
- congenital conditions.

Correlation between atrophic changes and clinical features is often poor.

Radiological features

- Irreversible loss of brain substance results in enlargement of the CSF spaces: the ventricles, basal cisterns, cerebral and cerebellar sulci. Ventricular dilatation may also be noted in hydrocephalus. However, in hydrocephalus, the ventricles dilate with relatively normal sulci, whereas in atrophy, there is usually both ventricular and sulcal enlargement.
- *Alzheimer's disease*: usually diffuse atrophy with relative sparing of the cerebellum; the temporal lobes may be severely affected.
- *Pick's disease*: circumscribed lobar atrophy.
- *Other dementias*: usually non-specific diffuse atrophy as in Alzheimer's disease.

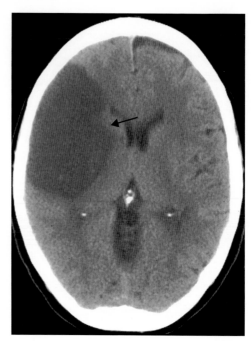

Figure 11.23 CT brain: recent middle cerebral artery territory infarct (arrow) showing a little mass effect with compression of lateral ventricle.

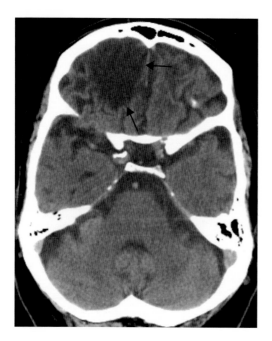

Figure 11.22 CT brain: anterior cerebral artery infarct to involve the frontal lobe (arrows).

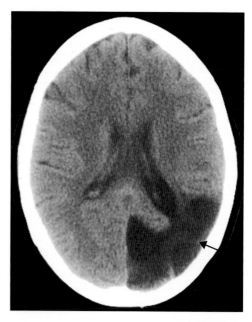

Figure 11.24 CT brain: well-established old posterior cerebral artery territory infarct (arrow).

Cerebral infarct

Infarction of the brain results from a deficient cerebral circulation from thrombosis or an embolic event and clinically presents as a stroke. Predisposing factors include a family history, hypertension, diabetes and the many causes of atherosclerotic disease or emboli. Symptoms and signs vary depending on the site of infarction.

- A transient ischaemic attack (TIA) produces a focal neurological deficit in which complete recovery of function occurs within 24 hours.
- A stroke is one in which the neurological deficit persists.

Radiological investigations

- CT/MRI of brain.
- Carotid artery imaging: magnetic resonance angiography (MRA)/Doppler ultrasound.
- Invasive arteriography should be avoided, but will occasionally be necessary.

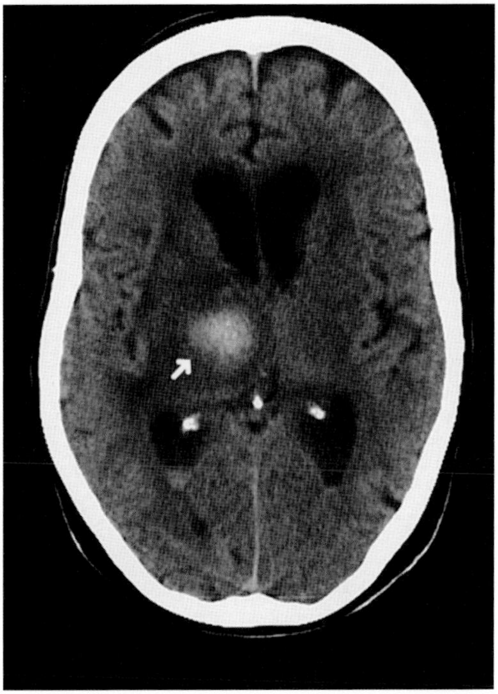

Figure 11.25 CT scan: haemorrhagic middle-cerebral artery infarct (arrow).

Radiological features

The most useful role of CT/MRI is to confirm the presence of an infarct and to exclude haemorrhage or other abnormalities, thus expediting treatment with aspirin or anticoagulants.

- *CT*: may be and remain entirely normal, but most substantial infarcts that are going to be seen are visible within the first 24 hours. Initial abnormalities are often subtle. Loss of grey/white matter differentiation evolves into reduced density, normally in an arterial supply territory, often with mild mass effect for the first few days and giving way to localized atrophic changes. About 15% develop haemorrhage, seen as an area of increased density.
- *MRI*: in association with MRA, is accurate and may demonstrate an occluded or stenosed vessel. The pattern and distribution of infarction are similar to CT.

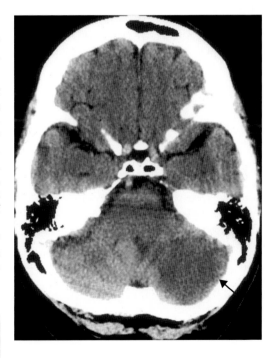

> **Key point**
>
> CT brain may be normal in an acute stroke for up to 24 hours

Figure 11.26 CT: cerebellar infarct (arrow).

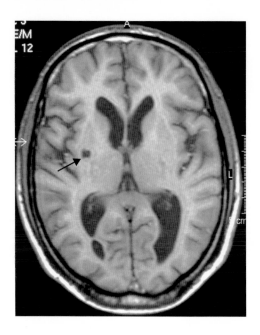

Figure 11.27 MRI: small lacunar infarct (arrow). Although the infarct is small it may, because of its position, have serious consequences.

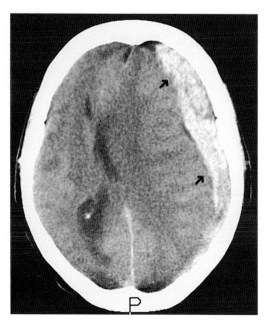

Figure 11.28 CT brain: recent subdural haematoma (arrows) with a significant midline shift.

Haemorrhagic infarct

About 5% of infarcts are associated with acute bleeding into the infarct. Diagnosis is important, because unlike the majority of ischaemic infarcts, anticoagulation is to be avoided in this group of patients.

Cerebellar infarct

Vertigo, loss of balance and diplopia are the principal signs of cerebellar infarction, seen as a focal area of low density on CT.

Lacunar infarct

A lacunar infarct occurs as a result of occlusion of small distal intracerebral arteries, they are usually less than 1 cm in diameter, in the region of the internal capsule, basal ganglia, thalamus and pons.

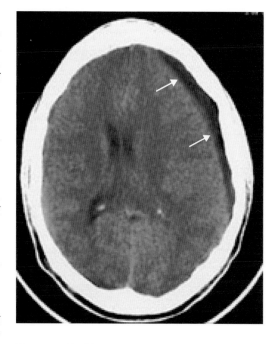

Figure 11.29 CT brain: old subdural haematoma showing low density (arrows).

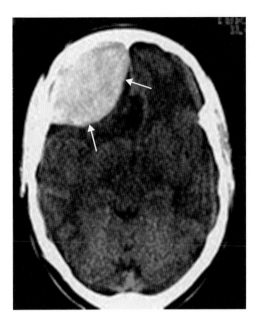

Figure 11.30 CT brain showing large right extradural collection with a convex inner border (arrows).

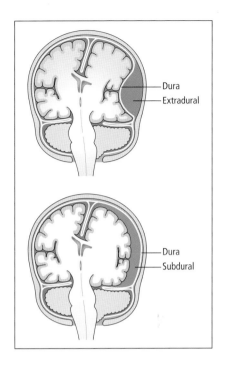

Figure 11.31 Intracranial haemorrhage.

Subdural haemorrhage

- A subdural collection initially shows an area of peripherally placed crescentic fluid collection, lying adjacent to the cranial vault.
- A recent haemorrhage is visualized as increased density (white), but subsequently this decreases to finally appear as an area of low density (black).
- Mass effect, with midline shift, indicates a significant subdural.
- Chronic subdural haematoma may be found in the elderly, with blood accumulating slowly in the subdural space, possibly from a ruptured vein.

Extradural haemorrhage

- Usually follows trauma and commonly associated with calvarial fractures.
- Laceration of the middle meningeal artery is the most common aetiology.
- Blood accumulates in the potential space between the dura and cranium.
- The classic lucid interval occurs in 20–50% of patients.
- Extradural haematoma has a convex inner border.
- Rarely extends beyond the sutures.

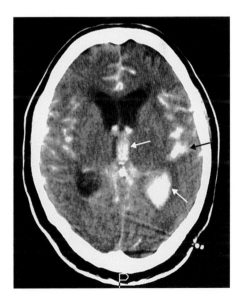

Figure 11.32 CT brain: subarachnoid haemorrhage with blood in the sulci, third ventricle and the posterior horn of the left lateral ventricle (arrows).

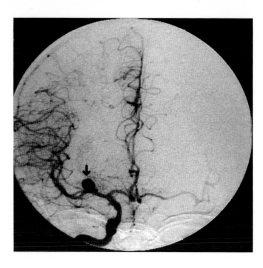

Figure 11.33 Arteriogram: aneurysm of the right middle cerebral artery (arrow).

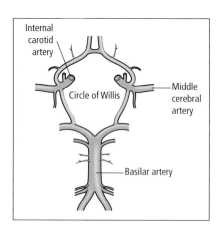

Figure 11.34 Circle of Willis.

Subarachnoid haemorrhage

A subarachnoid haemorrhage, usually spontaneous, occurs when there is bleeding into the subarachnoid space, between the arachnoid membrane and the pia mater surrounding the brain.

Presentation

- Sudden headache.
- Nausea and vomiting.
- Loss of consciousness.
- Convulsions.

Causes

- Spontaneous.
- Ruptured aneurysm, commonest cause.
- Trauma.
- Anticoagulant therapy.

Radiological features

- CT scanning is the investigation of choice, detecting recent blood in the cisterns, fissures or ventricles.
- Arteriography in spontaneous subarachnoid haemorrhage to detect source and site of bleeding – if suitable for surgical intervention.
- Intracranial aneurysms are discovered in approximately 70% of cases. Unruptured aneurysms of 4–5 mm are often not operated on unless shown to enlarge on interval imaging.

Complications

Hydrocephalus, either obstructive or communicating.

> **Key point**
>
> CT brain is normal in suspected subarachnoid haemorrhage, it is important to perform a lumbar puncture

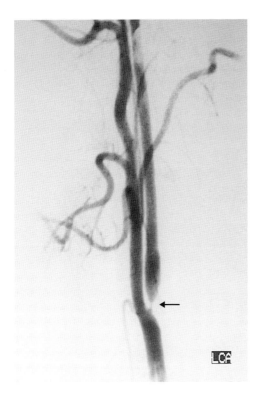

Figure 11.35 Arteriogram demonstrating a critical stenosis at the origin of the left internal carotid artery (arrow).

Carotid artery stenosis

Internal carotid artery stenosis may be either asymptomatic, present with transient ischaemic attacks (TIAs) or a stroke. In 30–40% of patients with TIAs, progression to a stroke results from distal infarction or embolization. The carotid artery may, however, occlude totally without causing any symptoms.

Radiological investigations

Colour Doppler ultrasound; arteriography.

Radiological features

- *Colour Doppler* accurately defines the stenosis, blood flow characteristics and alteration in peak velocities.
- *MRA* delineates the carotid arteries and any associated stenoses without the use of contrast material.
- *Arteriography*, readily shows the anatomical abnormality, but should be reserved for equivocal cases because of the risk of serious complications. The stenosis is usually found at the origin of the internal carotid artery.

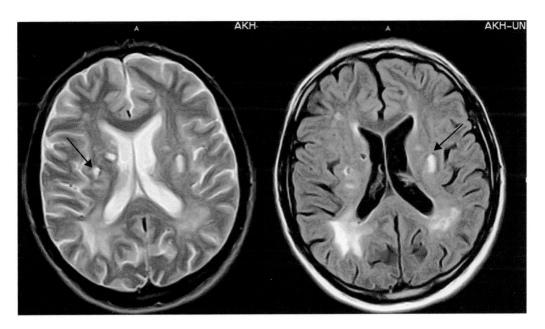

Figure 11.36 MRI scan with T1 and T2 sequences showing demyelination plaques (arrows) in the periventricular region.

Multiple sclerosis

Multiple sclerosis is a common neurological condition of young people, resulting in areas of demyelination in the central nervous system; it is of an unknown aetiology, more common in women, with a characteristic relapsing and remitting course of various neurological symptoms, depending on the site of the demyelinating lesions.

Radiological features

- CT is not accurate but may show atrophic brain changes in late disease.
- MRI is the investigation of choice and will confirm the disease by the presence of increased signal plaques in the periventricular deep white matter on the T2 sequence.
- Lesions may be seen in the spinal cord, optic nerves, brain stem or any other area of the CNS.
- Contrast enhancement of the plaques is indicative of active disease.

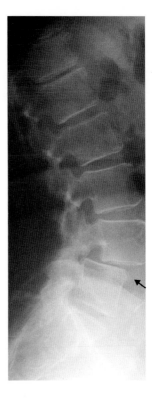

Figure 11.38 Spondylolisthesis at L4/L5 (arrow).

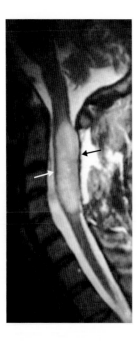

Figure 11.37 MRI cervical spine showing a large spinal cord glioma (arrows).

Spinal cord tumour

Spinal cord tumours may be any of the following.

- Metastases to the spinal cord from tumours outside the CNS.
- Metastases from seeding of intracranial neoplasms.
- Primary benign tumours, the most common being meningioma in the thoracic region.
- Primary malignant tumours – gliomas such as ependymoma or astrocytoma.

Radiological features

MRI is the primary imaging modality:

- expansion of the cord;
- reduction of CSF space around the tumour;
- focal mass, often cystic.

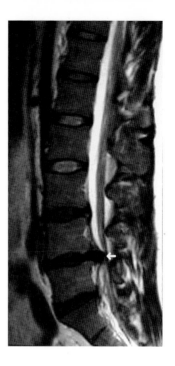

Figure 11.39 MRI scan demonstrating a prolapsed disc at L4/L5 with posterior deviation of the theca (arrow).

Spondylolisthesis

Spondylolisthesis refers to a slip of one vertebra on another, usually forwards but it may occasionally be backwards. It may be degenerative (associated with severe osteoarthritis of the posterior facet joints, usually L4/L5), congenital or post-traumatic, resulting in a defect in the pars interarticularis of the neural arch. It is often asymptomatic.

Radiological features

The slip is best demonstrated on a lateral projection of the lumbar spine and there may be an associated loss of disc space. The commonest affected levels are L4/L5 and L5/SI. CT/MRI evaluate the theca and any bony canal narrowing.

Treatment

- Conservative.
- Surgical: for a severe slip, internal fixation stabilizes the vertebra.

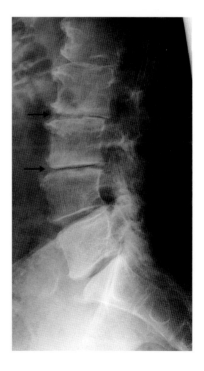

Figure 11.40 Typical degenerative changes in the lumbar spine with disc space narrowing (arrows).

Disc prolapse

Cervical spine

- Herniation of a central disk in the cervicothoracic region results in myelopathy with paraparesis, spasticity, hyperreflexia, clonus, sensory disturbance in the legs and sphincter dysfunction.
- With herniation of a high cervical central disk, respiratory compromise may occur.

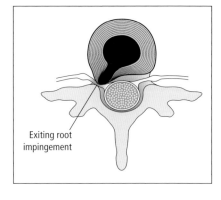

Figure 11.41 Right postero-lateral disc prolapse.

Thoracic spine

Thoracic disc herniations are rare.

Lumbar spine

- Most common site of disc herniation.
- L4/L5 prolapse (20% of cases): compression of the L5 root may result in foot drop and sensory loss of the outer aspect of the leg.
- L5/SI prolapse (70% of cases): SI root compression may cause an absent ankle jerk, with tingling and loss of sensation at the outer aspect of the foot.

Radiological features

- *Plain films.* Disc space narrowing, often with osteophyte formation, is best seen in the lateral projection.
- *MRI.* The investigation of choice for the accurate diagnosis of degenerative discs and disc prolapse or protrusion. However, degenerative disc disease is extremely common and must be correlated with clinical symptoms.
- *CT.* Demonstrates hypertrophic degenerative changes in the facet joints which may cause bony canal stenosis.
- *Myelography.* Now rarely performed. Injection of contrast into the spinal theca via a lumbar puncture to visualize the disc impression on the theca.

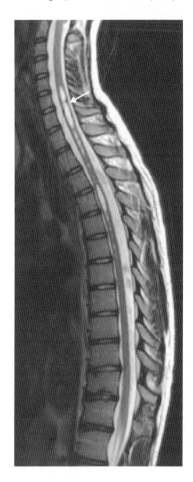

Figure 11.42 MRI cervical spine: fluid-filled central cord cavity in syringomyelia (arrow).

Syringomyelia

Syringomyelia refers to a cavity within the spinal cord often communicating with the central canal; it is most commonly found in the cervical cord and when it extends to the brain stem, it is called syringobulbia. Pain and temperature pathways are interrupted and may give rise to neuropathic joints.

Radiological features

MRI will readily reveal the central, fluid-filled cavity.

Causes

- Congenital: associated with the Chiari malformation.
- Post-traumatic; after spinal cord injury.
- Postinflammatory; following infections and subarachnoid haemorrhage.

12

Specific radiological investigations

Respiratory tract

Bronchial carcinoma

- Possibility of a bronchial carcinoma is usually raised following a chest X-ray, either from detecting a focal opacity, persistent consolidation or a lobar collapse.
- Computed tomography (CT) evaluates the mass and any associated mediastinal lymph node enlargement to assess operability of the tumour and also as a baseline study to follow progress after radiotherapy and chemotherapy.
- Positron emission tomography (PET) scanning will be helpful in establishing the presence of malignant spread to the nodes.
- Magnetic resonance imaging (MRI) is occasionally utilized to assess mediastinal or chest wall involvement. Small nodes, less than 1 cm in diameter, may be due to reactive hyperplasia rather than neoplastic infiltration.
- In peripheral lesions, a percutaneous lung biopsy is indicated if bronchoscopy is unable to yield a suitable specimen for histology.

Multiple lung metastases

- Pulmonary metastases are common from breast, colorectal and prostate cancer and occur with tumours that have rich systemic venous drainage – renal cancer, melanoma, testicular, thyroid and bone sarcomas.
- CT is considerably more accurate at detecting secondary deposits than a chest X-ray and will visualize metastases as small as 1 mm.

- CT thorax is required in patients with cancer as their detection will have a significant effect on patient management.

Cardiovascular system

Deep vein thrombosis

- Diagnosis is by colour Doppler ultrasound.
- Doppler scanning is non-invasive and readily available.
- Difficulty may be encountered in large limbs with poor visualization of the calf veins.
- Venography, with contrast injection into a foot vein, can be performed to accurately delineate thrombus, but this technique is now rarely used.

Pulmonary embolus

- A plain chest film may be entirely normal or show some non-specific signs, such as a pleural effusion or linear atelectasis.
- Ventilation/perfusion scans are moderately accurate for diagnosis but radiation dose is less than a CT.
- Contrast-enhanced CT of the pulmonary arteries is a rapid and accurate method of diagnosis and this is often the primary modality for evaluation of suspected pulmonary embolus.
- The invasive technique of pulmonary angiography with contrast injection directly into the pulmonary arteries is now rarely utilized, but this technique is occasionally used to disperse large life-threatening emboli in the main pulmonary arteries.

Radiology: Lecture Notes, Fourth Edition. Pradip R. Patel.
© 2020 John Wiley & Sons Ltd. Published 2020 by John Wiley & Sons Ltd.
Companion website: www.wiley.com/go/patel/radiology

Aortic aneurysm

- Ultrasound is simple and efficient as a screening tool for the detection of an aneurysm and following up abdominal aneurysms.
- Arteriography may determine the origin of the aneurysm and demonstrate the peripheral circulation.
- CT/MRI is required for suspected aortic dissection or a leaking aortic aneurysm.
- CT will accurately assess the extent of an aneurysm and its relationship to major arteries prior to treatment.

Stroke

- CT scanning may be normal up to 24 hours after the event.
- A haemorrhagic component appears as an area of high density.
- Early scanning is essential if thrombolysis is to be considered, as haemorrhage is a contraindication.
- Doppler ultrasound of the carotid arteries will assess stenoses.
- MRI of the carotid arteries and intracranial circulation will further assess the carotids and intracranial circulation.

Hypertension

- Onset of hypertension at a young age needs further investigation to discover a potentially curable cause, such as adrenal tumour or renal artery stenosis.
- Ultrasonography, isotope studies and CT may all detect a renovascular cause.
- MRI is now the best initial technique to look at the renal arteries.
- For inadequate studies, anatomical visualization by angiography still remains the definitive investigation.

Gastrointestinal tract

Dysphagia

- A barium swallow is the investigation of choice and often performed prior to endoscopy to avert the danger of perforation from conditions such as a pharyngeal pouch.
- A suspected leak or perforation is investigated by means of water-soluble contrast agents.

- In patients in whom aspiration is a possibility, gastrografin is contraindicated, as this particular contrast agent in the lungs can cause severe pulmonary oedema.

Change in bowel habit

- Colonoscopy is the investigation of choice. It is an accurate technique but may prove difficult in a tortuous colon with multiple redundant loops.
- CT colonography is also a reliable method of detecting colonic pathology. If a colonic carcinoma is discovered, abdominal CT will stage the tumour (para-aortic lymphadenopathy and liver metastases).
- Barium enema examination is now rarely utilized.

Gastrointestinal bleeding

Acute bleeding

- Isotope scans may detect bleeding rates as low as 0.1 ml/min.
- Arteriography is less sensitive and requires at least 0.5–1 ml/min but it may locate the exact site of haemorrhage for infusion of vasoconstrictors or embolization.
- Further evaluation of the small and large bowel can be carried out either by barium studies of the small bowel or colonoscopy of the large bowel.

Chronic bleeding

- Colonoscopy will visualize tumours.
- Arteriography has a low success rate in detecting lesions but may uncover tumours or angiodysplasia.
- Rarely, bleeding may be from a Meckel's diverticulum, when an isotope scan may detect ectopic gastric mucosa.

Abdominal mass

- Ultrasound will identify the cause of most abdominal masses, for example those in the liver, pancreas, kidneys or pelvis.
- Bowel masses may be difficult to visualize and require colonoscopy.
- CT is very useful for the evaluation of the origin of an abdominal mass, its surrounding relationships and to determine local or distant spread.

Biliary tract

Jaundice

- Ultrasound readily distinguishes an obstructive from a non-obstructive pattern by virtue of biliary duct dilatation and often confirms the level of obstruction.
- Endoscopic retrograde cholangiopancreatography (ERCP) will locate the site and often the cause of obstruction; common bile duct calculi can be removed at the same time.
- Magnetic resonance cholangiopancreatography (MRCP) is a successful MRI imaging technique for the visualization of the biliary tree.
- If ERCP is not technically successful, a transhepatic cholangiogram will provide similar information on the state of the biliary system; CT may be necessary for a suspected pancreatic tumour.

Acute pancreatitis

- Ultrasound may show a pleural effusion, enlargement of the pancreas and collections or pseudocysts.
- Ultrasound will accurately diagnose common bile duct dilatation and gallstones, an important cause of pancreatitis. However, bowel gas often precludes optimum visualization.
- CT is superior to ultrasound in demonstrating peripancreatic inflammatory changes and the presence of an abscess.
- Intravenous contrast enhancement provides valuable evidence of necrotic non-viable areas of the pancreas.

Chronic pancreatitis

- A plain abdominal film showing pancreatic calcification is virtually pathognomonic of chronic pancreatitis.
- Calcification and abnormal glandular structure can be readily detected by ultrasound and CT.
- ERCP confirms the state of the main pancreatic duct and its radicles.

Hepatosplenomegaly

- Good-quality plain films may show enlargement of the soft tissue shadows of the liver and spleen.

- Ultrasound, however, is the more appropriate investigation to confirm liver or splenic enlargement.

Liver metastases

- Ultrasound is a good initial investigation and will detect most metastases. It is also valuable as a screening test for patients with neoplastic disease.
- CT is the most sensitive and will also evaluate the rest of the abdomen, but will need a bolus of contrast injection.
- MRI is also accurate in localizing secondary deposits; arteriography is rarely necessary.

Urinary tract

Haematuria

- Principal initial investigations are ultrasound and CT urography.
- Ultrasound visualizes renal tumours, renal calculi, bladder tumours and prostatic enlargement.
- In haematuria, cystoscopy must always be performed even when all radiological investigations are normal.

Renal mass

- Ultrasound will readily identify the size, shape and nature of a renal mass.
- The vast majority are found to be simple cysts and appear as well-defined, echo-free lesions not needing any follow-up.
- If a mass is found to be solid, CT may ascertain the nature of the mass and assess local and distant spread.

Chronic renal failure

- Ultrasound is the screening procedure of choice in renal failure.
- Ultrasound assesses the size of kidneys and their appearance and identifies renal parenchymal disease.
- Ultrasound also detects the presence of renal obstruction and often its cause, such as renal calculi, pelvic malignancy or bladder outlet obstruction (most commonly due to prostatic enlargement).

Urinary tract infection

- Urinary tract infections are common in women.
- In males, even a single episode of infection requires further investigation.
- In children, micturating cystography either under fluoroscopy or by radionuclide studies will exclude the presence of vesico-ureteric reflux. Ultrasound detects any underlying congenital renal abnormalities or focal areas of renal scarring.

Renal tract obstruction

- Renal tract obstruction can occur in any part of the urinary tract but commonly results from pelvi-ureteric junction obstruction, ureteric calculus or bladder outlet obstruction.
- Calyceal or renal pelvic dilatation is easily demonstrated on ultrasound, though ureteric dilatation is not seen until a late stage.
- The commonest clinical problem is a ureteric calculus and ultrasound may demonstrate pelvicalyceal dilatation but will not determine the site of obstruction.
- A CT scan of the kidneys, ureter and bladder (CT KUB) will accurately localize the site of a ureteric calculus and demonstrate renal calculi.

13

Image viewing hints

Film-viewing hints

At some stage in your medical career, you will be asked your opinion on a radiological examination; this may be in the final medical examination, on ward rounds, at conferences or in postgraduate examinations. Efficient presentation will create a good overall impression to an accompanying clinical case.

There is no substitute for having previously studied and analysed a large number of images, as a fairly substantial part of radiology involves pattern recognition. There is no easy solution, and developing the ability for correct interpretation is a long-term process. It is important, therefore, in your clinical years, to be aware of the images that are associated with patient management and to attempt to look at and analyse them, if necessary in conjunction with the radiologist's report.

If you need some formal tuition, persuade a radiologist to show you some common conditions. It is important to specify that you want teaching on common conditions, as the radiologist's collection will often be full of rare and obscure cases. You need to see cardiac failure, gallstones, pneumonia, etc., not Takayasu's arteritis, cysticercosis and aorto-enteric fistulae, however fascinating they may be.

The images shown in examinations are usually straightforward, dealing with common clinical problems. The majority are plain films, e.g. chest, abdomen, etc. Contrast examinations may include studies of the gastrointestinal, urinary or biliary system, etc. When these are shown, be aware that they can be reproduced in either a white format or one in which the contrast-filled structures (arteries, veins, bladder, gut, etc.) appear black. Ultrasound, computed tomography (CT) and magnetic resonance imaging (MRI) are more advanced investigations but are becoming an integral part of patient investigation and a basic knowledge of these imaging modalities is required. You are less likely to be asked about their interpretation, except for the common pathologies on CT (liver metastases, renal calculi, fractures, lung carcinoma, etc.) and ultrasound (gallstones, liver abscess, etc.). You should know where these modalities fit in the sequence of investigating a patient. For example:

- jaundiced patient: ultrasound first, then CT, endoscopic retrograde cholangiopancreatography (ERCP) or CT;
- lung mass: plain chest X-ray, bronchoscopy, CT, percutaneous lung biopsy.

Begin talking within a few seconds of the image being displayed, and do not stay silent for longer than 10 seconds. It is better to start thinking aloud than to keep quiet: 'This is a chest X-ray and the lung fields appear clear. The cardiac shadow is normal in size and shape. Looking at the ribs …'. While you are describing this, you may come across an abnormal finding, or if you are fortunate, the examiner may interrupt with a helpful suggestion. If you do see an abnormality, don't feel you can relax; keep studying the image as there may be more than one abnormality. For example, if there is a lung mass, there may be an associated rib metastasis or pleural effusion. One or two pertinent questions are permissible, but no more. Remember that the examiners will generally be as helpful as they can. When commenting on an image, take it in logical steps, and do not jump from one to another. Each step should be completed before progressing to the next one.

- Identification of the image.
- Description of the abnormalities visible.
- Diagnosis or a differential diagnosis.

Identification of the image

Start by identifying the type of image presented to you. This might not be as simple as it seems. Plain films present no real problems, but contrast examinations may give rise to some difficulty.

Radiology: Lecture Notes, Fourth Edition. Pradip R. Patel.
© 2020 John Wiley & Sons Ltd. Published 2020 by John Wiley & Sons Ltd.
Companion website: www.wiley.com/go/patel/radiology

The image may be approached in a technically cor-rect manner: 'This is a chest X-ray taken in the posteroanterior projection. It is well penetrated and centred ...'. However, this often produces a lengthy introduction and an acceptable alternative practice is to eliminate many of the preliminaries and proceed straight to the film: 'This is a chest X-ray showing ...' or 'This is an abdominal X-ray showing ...'.

If a contrast examination is shown, of the bile ducts say, and you do not know whether it is a transhepatic, T-tube or a peroperative cholangiogram, a sensible approach to use would be to describe it initially as a contrast examination showing the bile ducts, or simi-larly: 'This is a contrast examination showing the large bowel ...' or 'This is a contrast examination showing the bladder ...', and then later try to ascertain the exact nature of the investigation.

Make a quick mental note of the name, if it is visible, as this may be important: first, to distinguish between a male and female patient; and second, to elucidate the ethnic origin, as both of these may give a clue to diag-nosis. If there is a particular area or abnormality that needs to be specified, identify it or point to it precisely.

Description

This should be short and succinct. Avoid giving lengthy, verbose descriptions as the aim is to reach a conclusion. Concentrate on the major abnormality: in describing a chest X-ray with a lung mass, do not start talking about the heart size, ribs, etc., and leave the description of the mass to the last. The examiner may think that you have not seen the abnormality. Describe the mass first, and while you are doing this, look for any other abnormality. If you do not see any, come to a diagnosis or a differential diagnosis.

Examiners will often give leading clues during the description, so take these gratefully. Remain calm and collected. If halfway through you realize that you are completely on the wrong track, or see something that contradicts your earlier description, do not strug-gle on. In this situation, it is reasonable to retract your statement and start all over again.

When viewing an image, for example a chest X-ray, you may need a lateral, or in the case of a contrast film, a control or preliminary film so it is permissible to ask if any further views are available.

Diagnosis or differential diagnosis

Only a few conditions will have a definitive or une-quivocal diagnosis, for example pneumothorax or emphysema; most have a differential diagnosis. Remember the common conditions. It is important in a differential to mention the commonest disor-ders first and relegate the rarer ones to the bottom of the list. Neoplasm should head the list of a solitary lesion in the lung, not hamartoma or hydatid cyst.

Leave some room for manoeuvre, and unless you are sure, do not reach a definitive diagnosis, as several answers are often possible. Most cases of image interpretation will usually have a differential diagnosis.

Typical examples of film description

Lung mass

This is a chest X-ray showing a well-defined opacity in the right upper zone. There is no calcification or cavitation associated with it. The appearances sug-gest a mass lesion and it is likely to be a neoplasm, either a primary or secondary. The differential diag-nosis would also include other causes of a solitary lung opacity, such as hamartoma, granuloma arterio-venous malformation, etc.

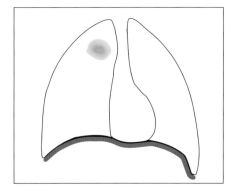

Cardiac enlargement, pericardial effusion

This is a chest X-ray showing a significantly enlarged cardiac shadow. The lungs show no abnormality. Causes of cardiomegaly would include cardiomyopathy, ischaemic heart disease and multiple valvular disease, but in view of the clear lung fields, the possibility of a pericardial effusion should be considered. An ultrasound examination will confirm this.

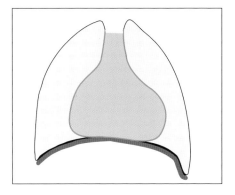

Oesophageal stricture

This examination is a barium swallow demonstrating narrowing in the lower oesophagus. There is mucosal irregularity associated with the narrowing and oesophageal carcinoma must be excluded. Secondary invasion from mediastinal tumours can also give rise to this appearance. The features are unlikely to be due to a benign stricture. An endoscopy with biopsy is necessary.

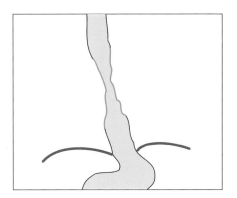

Gall stones

There are multiple opacities in the right hypochondrium on this plain abdominal film. These appear to be faceted and have the typical appearance of gall stones, but an ultrasound examination will readily confirm this.

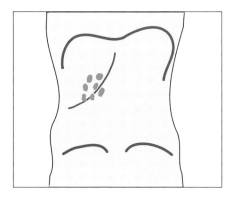

Ureteric calculus

The CT urogram shows distension of the left pelvicalyceal system. The ureter is dilated down to the level of the sacro-iliac joint and the appearances suggest obstruction. A pre-contrast CT may demonstrate a calculus in this region.

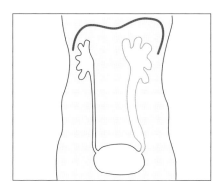

Osteoarthritis

This X-ray of the pelvis shows narrowing of the joint space at the right hip with osteophyte formation and articular irregularity. These are typical appearances of degenerative change.

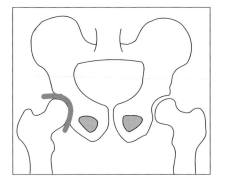

Cerebral infarct

This brain scan shows a low-density area in the right parietal lobe. There is a mass effect with midline shift and compression of the right lateral ventricle. The appearances are likely to be due to a recent infarct in the middle cerebral artery territory.

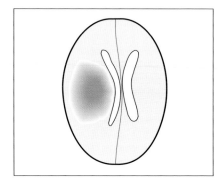

Index

Page numbers in *italics* refer to illustrations

Radiology: Lecture Notes, Fourth Edition. Pradip R. Patel.
© 2020 John Wiley & Sons Ltd. Published 2020 by John Wiley & Sons Ltd.
Companion website: www.wiley.com/go/patel/radiology